Nutrition's Playground

It's all about food in a roundabout way

By
Ben Pratt

Nutrition's Playground

First published in the United Kingdom by Natural Food Finder, www.naturalfoodfinder.co.uk

2 Hawthorn Way
Sawtry
PE28 5QB, UK

ISBN: 978-0-9568145-0-0

Cover design by Simon Norton
Printed and bound in Great Britain by
CPI Antony Rowe, Chippenham and Eastbourne

Nutrition's Playground

This book is dedicated to my wife, Rachael who has stuck by me through all the ups and downs that life throws at us. She has supported me over many years whilst together with our children we made a significant transition in our diet and witnessed firsthand the improved health and vitality it brought us.

Thank you.

Nutrition's Playground

Nutrition's Playground

Nutrition's Playground

Introduction: The Playground

The purpose and intention of this book is to discover, explore and reveal essential truths about food that are rarely understood. Current eating habits have led us to a point of widespread obesity and ill health, whilst the true principles for achieving optimal health and wellbeing have been known and applied for generations. It is our modern way of life that has blinded us with technology and science and along the way allowed our focus to be drawn away from these inherent, natural truths. Knowing what is right is only part of the battle. This book will also arm you with real solutions and motivational techniques that will ensure you follow through and make your goals of optimal health and weight a reality. However, before we rush headlong into our exploration of myths and truths, I want to share a story in preparation for applying the truths to be learned on this journey.

Life has a wonderful way of providing us with beautiful highs and contrastingly difficult lows. Childhood is often full of many happy and exciting memories that we sometimes lose an appreciation of as we get older and familiarity steals the rush. Clear your mind. Focus your attention on this scene and draw on your own memory and experience.

Remember your home when you were a child, the walls, the smell, the sounds of family life, the laughter and love you felt from those around you. Outside it is summer time; the sun is beaming down bringing warmth and life to the back garden.

Nutrition's Playground

The lure of the outside for a child is almost unbearable, but mum has promised you a trip to the park after lunch. You are already getting impatient, it seems likes ages ago since you finished lunch and clambered down from the table. You have had your shoes on and been gazing out the back door for what seems an eternity, while the sounds of mum cleaning the dishes is the only thing breaking what would otherwise be silence. Your mind is ahead of reality and you are already there, running around in the sun, swinging, sliding, laughing and riding the waves of happiness and excitement that only a child knows.

Suddenly silence! The tap has stopped! You hear mum's footsteps and the words you have been waiting to here, "Come on then, let's go." A huge smile breaks out across your face and your heartbeat jumps up a gear. At last! You can't stand still as you wait for mum to unlock the door. You know the way to the local park like the back of your hand, but mum agonisingly asks you to stay nearby. With each step along the footpath your excitement seems to step up a little too. As you hold mums soft, but safe hands you keep looking for the usual point where she says you can run on ahead. There it is at the end of the path, the entrance to the open expanse of parkland. Mum hasn't let go yet, but you can just make out the yells and laughter of other children playing being carried by the cool summer breeze. You can feel the warmth and smell of the country as your senses are enlivened by that summer something that is hard to put your finger on. You feel her grip ease and mum gently encourages you on, the adrenaline surges and you break out into a run. The field opens out before you and not too far away the bright red, blue and yellow paint of playground apparatus sparkles in the sun. The grass gently slopes down and as you run you can hardly keep up with your own feet as you keep trying to run a fraction quicker than you actually are able. You keep your gaze fixed on the equipment you want to play on first, the climbing frame.

Apparatus

You wrap your fingers tightly round the lower rungs and pull your weight upwards seeking to reach the heights that this mountain of a structure offers. With practise you have learned to keep as many limbs in contact as possible to prevent slipping. Going higher than the other children you have overcome your early fears and reach the pinnacle of the climbing frame, a place where only the bravest children go! This is a great place to be, where you can look out with pride at the other children playing and as you catch your mum's gaze she smiles proudly at your achievement. There is something satisfying about overcoming even imaginary mountains to gain the perspective that can only be seen from the top. However, the climbing frame does have one drawback, once you have reached the top there is nowhere else to go! The only option is to clamber back down and try another of the playgrounds attractions.

The swing is a long time favourite that is present in just about every playground across the country. You rush over perch onto the seat then call over to mum to come and push you, after all its always better when someone is there to get you started, then you just work to maintain the momentum. After a few swift pushes from mum she leaves you to carry on. Leaning back to drive your feet skyward you are soon soaring through the air, the wind rushing past a subtle reminder of the rush it is to momentarily beat gravity as you swing upwards. The sun causes you to squint each time it shines in your face as your reach the forward, upper most apex of the swing. In that moment you almost wish you could bottle up how you feel to be exhilarated through the movement

Nutrition's Playground

experienced by something as simple as a swing. With the sounds of the children beside you laughing and squealing with delight a basic physical lesson is learned. As soon as you stop working at maintaining the momentum you lose height and will soon return to a static position back at the starting point. The swing brings joyous highs but ultimately returns you back to the same place as soon as your effort dwindles.

As your swing slows you glance around deciding where to go next. Out of the corner of your eye you see a friend sat alone on the seesaw, you jump off the slowly moving swing and rush over offering to join in. Your friend smiles with delight and with a burst from your feet you are rocketed into the air with ease. At the top you briefly lift off your seat then swiftly drop back down to earth. You work together at alternating moments to keep the experience going responding to how hard each other has pushed off the ground. It's a much harsher, bumpier ride, but is great fun all the same. Another lesson is learned, what goes up must come down, and in this case if your partner doesn't take care you often descend with a crash!

In the midst of your fun a soft voice calls out your name. You recognise your mums tones and turn to see her motioning that it is time to go. You quickly bargain for one last turn on a key piece of apparatus that you haven't tried – the slide! It doesn't matter how many times you have made the trip to the park the slide is always a must. At the foot of the steps you look up the ladder counting each rung as you climb…8, 9, and 10! At the top you can see clear across the park and wave at mum on the other side. You sit; edge forward, then effortlessly let gravity take over as you whiz down to the bottom. There is something rewarding about applying a little effort on the climb to get a free ride back down. Back holding mums hand you are brightly smiling all the way across the parkland to the path you originally walked earlier that afternoon. Then just as you turn the corner you catch a last glance at the park, some children still playing, wondering how long it will be until mum brings you back.

It is wonderful to imagine, remember or visualise as it brings experiences much closer to our current reality. This simple task of creating or remembering a childhood experience at the park is much more than a trip down memory lane. It most likely evoked responses in you and stirred up fond emotions within. It teaches us a powerful lesson in how to motivate ourselves to achieve and do things we desire or have found difficult in the past. Thoughts, when consciously directed, stimulate emotion, which is a significantly more potent driving force to action than just a random thought or decision. Also the story itself serves as a very accurate analogy for the many different dietary habits that exist in current society and the relationships we harbour with food. This book seeks to not only explore current food habits, identifying myths and seeking out truths, but to provide real solutions that support you throughout your nutritional development. It is appropriate at this point to expand on the parallels the story draws with society's current dietary habits.

A walk in the park

Firstly let's discuss the young child stood at the door longing to be in the park, gazing out waiting for when it would be time. How often do we look at others, what they have or are what they are doing, longing to be like them, yet do nothing to bring it into our existence? Do we create our own imaginary glass door blocking our passage to the things we desire because somehow we feel we are powerless to obtain it? But just like the young child with the right assistance, mum opening the door, we are able to go outside and begin our journey. Perhaps it may require someone or something to remove the mental block that is stopping your progress so you can then choose to begin your journey to obtain your desires. In certain cases that someone may well be you! In other cases you may need to be ignited by another. My intention is that this book will be a significant motivator for you to start your journey and develop a positive, healthy relationship with nutrition.

The park itself is a great reflection of western views on food habits and dietary trends. Since the early 80's food marketing has become a very powerful force and greatly influences the general public's opinion of what is healthy and what is not. As obesity rates have increased the desire to lose weight has risen with it. This has been a golden nugget that food marketing could not resist. Today so much effort is placed on lowering fat in foods, lowering salt, lowering cholesterol, lowering sugar, encouraging weight loss, reducing body fat, building muscle, changing shape and basically looking better. This has brought about the introduction of many new products and foods that we have not previously had in our food chain. It has also stimulated the creation of a myriad of diets all claiming to be the next ultimate answer to the weight management equation! In my years of experience advising others on nutrition I have met client's who have tried most of the popular diets with varying levels of success. Each piece of apparatus in 'Nutrition's Playground' represents a different style or approach that has been implemented to achieve the seemingly unobtainable goal of ideal weight and optimal health. Although each of these analogies applies to dietary approaches I have had experience of I will not mention them by name, but just describe the characteristics, so that you may find similarities from your own experience.

Nutrition's Playground

The climbing frame requires strength, coordination and determination to reach the top, but once you are there you have nowhere else to go, you have reached the end. Some dietary approaches on the surface seem quite complex and require a great deal of determination to apply them to your life. You need to be organised and have strength of character to stick to the overwhelming list of do's and don'ts that need to be navigated around, just like the rungs and bars of the climbing frame. The 'never say die' attitudes of those who usually take on these complicated approaches often drive the dieter through to completion. But once you have got the hang of the rules, and the initial benefits have been obtained, the diet cannot take you anywhere else, you reach the end of your progression on your nutrition journey. There are no options or alternate routes. Just one set of rules for anyone who chooses to follow. These diets tend to have varying levels of success, for some they work well, but for others they never quite work out and are just too hard to maintain in combination with their current life and circumstances. Basically you are stuck at the top of the climbing frame. So your choice is continue to sit there doing the same old thing or climb back down and try something else.

With a little help from someone else to get started the swing is an exhilarating ride. Whilst you keep up the effort and momentum the ride continues to deliver an enjoyable experience. However, as soon as effort wanes momentum immediately slows and the ride is less interesting and grinds to a halt. Certain organisations rely on a group setting to stimulate motivation or accountability, depending on how you view it, to help kick-start some form of low calorie diet. Often friends are made within these groups, which plays a role in maintaining the momentum and enjoyment of the experience, whilst effort is being applied and success is being achieved. But like the swing when effort tires because the heights needed to keep achieving new targets become unrealistic, then momentum and results usually slow. Suddenly the group setting can become uncomfortable as you miss the targets set each week. As your swing slows down you may be keen to get out and jump off the swing before it has even stopped.

Unfortunately in these group settings the other members of the group can clearly see whether you are losing weight successfully or whether you have slowed down and are just sitting on a stationary swing. To add to the frustrating experience it is often the case that within a relatively short time after the low calorie diet has ceased, weight that was lost begins to creep back on. Then the real lesson of the swing approach becomes clear – you had fun for a while, but when you're done you have ended up right back where you started, back at your pre-diet weight! Unfortunately some people jump straight back on the swing for another ride hoping that a second stab at this dietary approach might prove to be more successful than the first. But it is impossible for a swing to take you to a different place. More times than not you will end up right back where you started!

The seesaw is an explosive ride, blasting you skywards with a rapid descent to follow. Some dietary methods promise huge success in a very short period of time, the marketing and dynamic advertising screaming at easy methods of success. Lose seven pounds in one week! Drop a dress size in two weeks! Lose 4 inches in ten days! These are claims that seem to cover the glossy magazines and tabloid newspapers week in week out, each one really after quick consumer interest to sell their wares, rather than long-term commitment to their methodology of success. However, the promise of instant results seems to be a powerful lure to many. The bigger the results and the simpler the method the more interest it

Nutrition's Playground

creates. Many of these programmes are a bit extreme in their approach and use clever ways of tricking the body for a short period of time. Often dehydration, loss of carbohydrate based glycogen stores, muscle mass loss and in some instances some minimal fat loss are the ways in which these diets 'appear' to provide quick weight loss and seemingly powerful results. The seesaw parallels ring loud and clear when after the initial effects that send your spirits skyward, gravity takes over and with a slightly harder 'bump' you return to earth and realise that the initially impressive results are very short lived! What goes up must come down after all. Quick, short lived changes are all these fad diets can ever really offer. What is really needed is long term, revitalising healthy habits and living.

The final playground apparatus is the slide. Every playground across the country has a slide. Why is this considered such an essential ride? How does climbing to the top of a ladder and sliding to the bottom provide such a thrill to so many children? Maybe it's because we spend our lives fighting against gravity and its relentless effects, and for a moment, just a few seconds, we can let gravity take over and simply flow with the sensations it creates. The nutritional analogy here is different. The slide firstly takes us to a different place! The other apparatus inevitably return you to the same place each and every time. There is work to be done to climb to the top of the slide and appreciate the heights and enhanced perspective that can be observed there. But the real joy, the reward for getting there is that there is a free ride waiting to take you to a new place! And this ride is always a fun and exciting experience!

The core of this book, the heart of the message of Nutrition's Playground is that successful, health promoting, energy providing; weight managing, enjoyable nutrition is directly analogous to a simple slide! Initially a certain amount of effort

Nutrition's Playground

will need to be applied to prepare, gain knowledge, plan your actions, break distractive habits, and create powerful new habits. In Nutrition's Playground the slide has ten steps, ten revealing chapters of understanding truth, obliterating myths and creating change. Once the groundwork has been laid and the rungs of the ladder climbed then, and only then, can the ride be thoroughly enjoyed as your body and life travel smoothly to a new rewarding and satisfying place! Whether this place is improved health, lasting energy and vitality, a happy relationship with food, successfully finding your body's ideal weight, or just the plain enjoyment of fantastic food the lesson is the same. The slide in Nutrition's Playground is the route that will deliver the answer. Not only is there modern science to back up many of the principles taught within these pages, but also years and generations of time tested, traditional nutrition secrets that are unlocked and revealed for your benefit. Your years of thrill seeking amongst the diet pages of modern magazines and books are over! This ride will provide the answer you have been seeking. So prepare for the rungs of the ladder, the work and effort lie ahead. Read, learn, apply and rest assured the slide will follow and the rewards will be worth all your effort and more.

Nutrition's Playground

Step 1: Short-sighted Convenience

The western world comprises Great Britain, the United States of America, Canada, France, Spain, Germany, Sweden, Europe as a whole, Japan, Australia and New Zealand. These are countries that we view as technologically advanced with all the wonders of the modern world! Yet amongst these modern countries we still find that many of their supposedly advanced inhabitants do not have the full measure of health that they ought to. Scientifically, we understand more now about nutrition than ever before! We have identified the macronutrients, fats, proteins and carbohydrates, as well as many hundreds of micronutrients, vitamins, minerals and phytochemicals. With all this knowledge why are we still finding many people each year struggling to reach a state of optimal health and others actually suffering from malnutrition? We know what vitamins do, what minerals can do, the effects of enzymes, bacteria, additives, preservatives, colours, flavourings, and other chemical concoctions! Science has studied and tracked their functions for generations now. Why then have we not been able to master the skill of keeping ourselves healthy?

Stark Stats

Statistics are often very revealing! They can provide us with a snap shot of truth that may have been difficult to be aware of without them. Let me identify just a few of the statistics from

Nutrition's Playground

the United Kingdom that may help us get an understanding of why Western health has become what it currently is.

One in every three Britons says that they do not eat vegetables because they require too much effort to prepare

In the year 2003 Britain ate more ready meals than the rest of Europe put together

In 2004 40% of British patients entering and leaving hospitals were found to have malnutrition

69% of Britons are still confused about which foods are healthy

Britain eats more than half of all crisps and savoury snacks eaten in the whole of Europe

(Blythman, 2006)

In the United Kingdom we don't eat vegetables very often! We love ready meals! Crisps are one of our favourite snacks! We struggle to even feed nutritious food to patients in hospital! Take a moment and think of all the traditional foods that you really love. What sorts of foodstuffs come to mind? Think of the food that you tucked into as a child, the flavours, the smells, the textures and the memories. I wonder what foods came to your mind. Steak and kidney pie? Fish and chips wrapped in newspaper? Instant trifle? Instant gravy? Condensed soup? Corned beef? Candyfloss? A stick of rock? The list could go on and on. But what is the common theme? We seem to have a love for industrialised food!

Nutrition's Playground

The supermarket's share

In the United Kingdom over 80% of all money spent on food is spent at the supermarket checkout (Blythman, 2004). Asda's Tesco's, Sainsbury's, Morrison's, Iceland, Budgen's, Marks and Spencer's and Waitrose are but a few of these institutions to which we have become so faithful. Is this a bad thing? Surely the supermarkets provide us with some convenience? There are usually several to choose from in each major town. More recently the supermarket is being morphed into smaller, local shops that provide even greater convenience to the residents of suburbs and housing estates. Supermarkets can only grow where there is demand after all. Back in the 1980s the supermarket was a relatively new force on the food front. The public was beginning to recognize the convenience that they provided and the benefits of finding everything they needed for their weekly shop in one place. There were only a limited number of products available on the shelves. In the 20 or 30 years since then, the variety of products available on the shelves has grown to more than 20,000 foodstuffs! We have choice beyond belief! And many of these products are centred on making our lives just that little bit more convenient. Western life is so fast paced, so hectic, so pressured, that people barely have time to think, never mind sit down and plan a decent meal. In order to keep up with this frantic ride some things need to be sacrificed. Often we may find that food is the casualty that gets left in the trenches to be dealt with only when circumstances allow. Food has become merely a fuel for the body; something that needs to be done to provide energy for all the other things that we want to do - a mere chore, a check box that needs to be ticked!

Let's take a moment just to analyse modern supermarket foods. A trip up and down the aisles of any supermarket can

Nutrition's Playground

begin to tell a story. Imagine your local supermarket, the familiar aisles, smells, sights and sounds. It's normally organised into beautiful departments. Fruit and vegetables, dairy, home-baked goods, ready meals, sandwich meats and cheeses, frozen foods, confectionery, alcohol, soft drinks, nuts, crackers, and crisps. Most of these foods are preserved in some way or other. Canning, drying, pickling, freezing, dehydrating, pasteurising, homogenising, and vacuum packing are a few of the many ways in which manufacturers strive to increase the shelf-life of their products. Why increase shelf life? It's simple business strategy. Decrease the amount of waste and subsequently increase sales and productivity! Another sneaky little benefit is most foodstuffs are packaged in boxes or containers. These serve as miniature billboards. They may not be adorned with flashing lights, but they catch your attention nonetheless and the attractive promise of what's inside adds to the irresistible lure that results in a purchase!

'Most marketing is spent on food with the lowest nutritional value'

There are literally thousands of new foods on our shelves. The shops we purchase food from are very different to how they used to be. So has food production remained unchanged? And the answer is emphatically no! The 20th century saw the rise of chemical farming. The use of fertilisers, pesticides and fungicides in food production has risen dramatically over the last 50 years, the harmful effects of which are beginning to become more obvious. Farmers have begun new intensive farming methods to maximise production in the shortest possible time. Animals are reared to adulthood in significantly less time with factory-like precision. Fields are mono-cropped for several years, leeching nutrients from the soil and causing the production of deficient grains and vegetable matter. This is a little bit like

20

using the same exercise programme again and again for months on end. At first the programme is fun and exciting and brings great results, but in time it becomes boring and dull and the initial results slow as the programme becomes stale. To get further results you have got to change the workout. A single crop in a field for years on end is like a dull, unchanging programme. Great results initially, followed by poor results later down the line.

It gets worse

The food chain is obviously not the only thing that has changed in the last 50 to 60 years. Technology has made life so much easier! We have all kinds of gadgetry that makes our physical activity levels significantly lower, from washing machines to vacuum cleaners and cars to remote controls. I can remember being at a friend's house observing a full 10 minute search for the remote control among the cushions of the sofa coupled with frustrated communications! It would have taken a matter of seconds to get off the chair and change the channel on the television! Perhaps that was just too much effort at the time. So nutrition is not the only change. Granted. But it's a big part of the equation

One result of these monumental changes in our food and activity levels is the rate that obesity is skyrocketing. We don't have the time to go into all countries in the Western world, but let's focus on the United States and the United Kingdom. In the United States from 1980 to 2008 obesity rates in adults aged 24 to 70 increased from 15% to a staggering 33.8%! (CDC, 2010) In the United Kingdom the rate of obesity has also increased rapidly reaching 24% for adult males and 25% for adult females in the year 2008 (HSE, 2010). Alarmingly this has virtually tripled since the early 1980s. So in both cases obesity has more than doubled within a 25-year period! If that trend carries on expert projections are suggesting a one in two obesity rate within the next 25 years.

Science has begun to recognize a new disease condition called metabolic syndrome. It was previously known as syndrome X. Scientists have found that a number of health disease risk factors generally occur together. These risk factors comprise:

- elevated blood pressure

- centrally occurring obesity

- insulin resistance (diabetic tendencies)

- increased blood clotting

- raised blood cholesterol

In scientific terms this is a relatively new discovery. It's only been in the last 20 years that the prevalence of these five conditions occurring together had become apparent to the medical community. It is difficult to know how many people in both the United Kingdom and the United States suffer from metabolic syndrome. However, estimates in both nations suggest that 25% of the population show clear signs of metabolic syndrome. That's one in four! Look back over those five conditions, and consider the strain on the health service caused by these five differing conditions. The time, money and focus spent on dealing with blood pressure, diabetic conditions, cholesterol problems and obesity runs into the billions of pounds or dollars. In the United Kingdom the taxpayer ultimately covers these costs. In the United States insurance companies pick up the bill, which clearly drives up the cost of insurance premiums.

Nutrition's Playground

Let me paint a picture for you of how health in the Western world has spiralled to the brink of control. When William Einthoven invented the electrocardiogram (ECG) in 1903 many critics suggested that he should have spent his time and effort doing something more worthwhile! This is because problems associated with heart disease were virtually unheard of. So although it was impressive to be able to measure the electrical activity of the heart, the medical establishment didn't really see the need for it. However, by 1924 Einthoven was given the Nobel Prize in medicine. Within a 20-year period that ECG machine had gained huge credibility because of the increased need or prevalence of associated problems of the heart. It is almost impossible today to see how the medical profession would be able to get by without the technology offered by the ECG machine.

Within the space of a single century cardiovascular disease has become one of the major killers in the world! Prior to this it was a virtually unheard of problem. This would suggest that we only need to investigate what has changed in the last 100 years to work out what the source of the problem is. But this is the age of technology and so much has changed. So how on earth are we supposed to know which areas to focus on? Is that not the point? Just like metabolic syndrome there are likely to be many factors that combine together to bring about the poor levels of health that we are witnessing today. Just like an avalanche starts with a small movement of snow and builds into something vastly destructive, the factors contributing to ill health have snowballed together and are careering down the mountainside of human health wiping out everything in their path. Just look at the major problems that exist. There is tooth decay and dental deformities, cardiovascular disease, diabetes, cancer, osteoporosis, arthritis, asthma, depression, a wide variety of learning difficulties and hormonal disruption. These more common conditions only represent the tip of the iceberg. Unfortunately it is not the most positive of pictures, is it?

Health hazard

In the United Kingdom the national budget for Healthcare services was set at £96 billion for the year 2006 - 2007! (HM Treasury, 22-03-2006). In the United States medical costs have been quoted as being as high as $2 trillion in 2007! (Associated Press, 2007). More money than ever before is being spent on medical care and health care! That is not just the result of an improvement in the health care system, but a reflection on the significant state of ill-health within the Western world. There are more significant and widespread health care problems now than perhaps at any time in history.

Imagine this situation. You've been to a shop and just purchased a 1000 piece jigsaw. You are a bit of the jigsaw buff after all. When you get home you eagerly open the box keen to get the first few pieces of the edging in place. But to your horror there are only 100 pieces in the box! What would you do? I can imagine you would take the box straight back to the shop and demand a replacement or your money back. After all you don't see much of the picture with only 100 out of 1000 pieces. The few pieces put together may give you some clues of what the picture actually is but the whole picture certainly cannot be seen.

Scientific research in many cases has become much like the scenario portrayed above. So often the efforts made are about trying to isolate individual chemicals or compounds that play a pivotal role in the removal of the disease or the regaining of our health. Medical science seems to spend so much effort in trying to find the magic pill, the ultimate answer. When we feel unwell the doctor provides some medication based on the signs and symptoms observed. This simplistic, allopathic approach may have some influence upon the illness at hand, but doesn't rebuild health from the ground up. If anything it may relieve some of the symptoms for a while, buying the doctor just a little bit more time. It's like expecting that 1000 piece jigsaw when only 100 pieces are available. It takes many nutrients and controlling mechanisms to bring body chemistry back into harmony. To achieve optimal health we need to be able to step away and observe the wonder of all the nutrients working together in the miracle that is the human body. Studying the heart by itself does not provide an appreciation of the working of the whole body.

Perhaps one of the most basic flaws in modern medicine is that much time is spent analysing and researching the sick in an attempt to understand how to be healthy! This approach surely is focused upon illness and understanding how illness and disease spreads throughout the body. An understanding of illness does not provide the complete picture of optimal health. Consider this. What would be the best way to learn how to use the latest computers on the market today? Understanding the various hardware components, the monitor, keyboard and internet router; the vast choice of software, which programmes were most reliable, keeping current with the latest versions and how to use all of the features to their greatest potential. There is also the speed at which technology is moving forward, processor speed, memory size, available RAM, broadband width, video streaming and web based media. This list of things seems endless. Would I be able to receive a full understanding of all these various factors if a specialist in anti-virus software had been solely responsible for my training? There is no doubt he would have an appreciation of some of these factors and could guide me on how to protect my computer from infection with suitable software and regular checking. It is

Nutrition's Playground

highly unlikely that he would be able to teach me all that would be needed to use the wide variety of other software and the latest technological developments! This is exactly what is going on in the modern medical model of health care. By relying on a myriad of medical specialists the focus is centred on dysfunctions of small parts of the body, but in so doing they are unable to understand the whole! True health must focus upon the complete body to be sure that each of the individual component parts are contributing to and serving the interests of the whole. Does this mean a complete 180 degree turn in health care? Perhaps not, but there is definitely a need for significant change. A better way to achieve optimal health would be to seek out and fully understand how the truly healthy people in the world live and what underpins the mastery of what today is such a rare condition.

'The key to real health is studying how the healthy have become so healthy, not why the unhealthy have become so unwell'

Modern eating habits and modern medicine seem to have one common feature. They are both focused on short term gain and providing the most convenient answer to fit in with the fast-paced, hectic lifestyles that have become such a prevalent part of modern living. Perhaps that is the real problem, our determination not to have time to care for our health properly!

Nutrition's Playground

Step 2: Traditional Human Health

" …since our orthodox theories have not saved us. We may have to re-adjust them to bring them into harmony with nature's laws. Nature must be obeyed, not orthodoxy. Apparently many primitive races have understood her language better than have our modernised groups. Even the primitive races share blights when they adopt our conception of nutrition."

Dr Weston A Price has been referred to as the 'Charles Darwin of nutrition.' He was born in 1870 and lived until 1948. He was a dentist by trade, and spent most of his days based in Cleveland, Ohio. Dr Price became increasingly concerned at the high level of dental cavities and deformed dental arches he was seeing day-to-day at his practice. He had heard stories of primitive people who reportedly had perfect teeth without the assistance of modern dentistry. This intrigued Dr Price, who chose to leave his practice for a time and venture out to seek these people. He wanted to know how they had obtained such wonderful dental health. During the 1920s and 30s, at their own expense Dr Price and his wife travelled to many places around the globe, identifying and studying the habits of untouched, indigenous human groups. He travelled to isolated villages in Switzerland, the Gaelic communities in the Outer Hebrides, the Eskimos and Indians of North America, the Melanesian and Polynesian South Sea

Nutrition's Playground

Islanders, a handful of African tribes, Australian aborigines, New Zealand Maori and the Indians of South America.

Dr Price was a meticulous scientist. As he worked amongst these primitive people he diligently documented literally thousands of teeth, noting down the rate and the incidence of dental cavities. This was not always easy, as Dr Price often had to observe various traditions and cultural etiquette in order to get the permission from the village or tribal chiefs and leaders. As well as documenting cavities Price also made fairly accurate records, considering his circumstances, of the foods that were being eaten by each primitive group. He took samples of the foods and sent them home to his laboratory for analysis. His purpose in taking such steps was to find out exactly what nutrients were contained in their traditional foods that brought about such marvellous health. Where possible, Dr Price also made enquiries about the health of the primitive cultures. Sometimes this was from the people themselves, whilst other times he obtained his information from pioneer and frontier doctors or missionaries in the area.

The timing of Price's travels couldn't have been better! Not only was he able to find these isolated primitive cultures and study their health, but in almost every case he was able to find and see the influence of Western foods amongst small portions of these people. It is unlikely that a similar study carried out today would be so successful at locating isolated populations with a mild influence of Western civilisation. Dr Price's work has been referred to and quoted by many health professionals across several generations. Robert Cathcart M.D. said that Price's work was:

'a must for anyone seriously interested in the effects of food on health.'

Nutrition's Playground

As Dr Price was one of the foremost nutrition pioneers in our day, it is worth taking a little bit more time to fully appreciate and understand the work that he did. There isn't the time to look through all the population groups that Price investigated, but it is worth looking through three or four adult population groups to widen and broaden our understanding of his pivotal discoveries.

Traditional travels

In Weston Price's outstanding book, Nutrition and Physical Degeneration, he first documented his journey to Switzerland, in particular to a valley high in the mountains called the Loeschental Valley. These wonderful people were, many miles from the influence of Western culture. There was no influence of commerce or medicine. These people were fantastically healthy and thrived in their remote environment. The people lived in a number of small villages that dotted the lush green valley. The Catholic Church had influenced the people creating a real desire for education. This had resulted in children being schooled for six months of the year, and then having the remaining six months to help with the farming. The Swiss were particularly keen on raising cattle on the lush, rapidly growing green grass that was primarily responsible for sustaining the whole ecosystem and culture of the people. Dairy produce, and rye used to make sourdough bread were the staple foods amongst these traditional living people. In particular the butter that was produced in early spring from the rapidly growing spring grass was highly prized and considered a sacred food.

Weston Price documented that the average number of dental cavities per person was 0.3. In other words, he found a cavity only once in every three or four people. In today's world it is more likely that to find a cavity in every three or four teeth! If

Nutrition's Playground

it isn't surprising enough to find such amazing dental health where no dentists lived, there were absolutely no documented cases of tuberculosis in the whole valley! This might not seem like such a big deal when there were only 2000 people living in the valley. Tuberculosis at the turn-of-the-century was a major problem in the Western world. The health of these people in general, was nothing short of amazing. Remember they were living in a remote mountain valley, with but a small mountain pass providing access. They could only live off exactly what was in that valley. They relied heavily on the unpasteurised milk from their herd of cattle. Tuberculosis was at the time thought to have come predominantly from tainted unpasteurised milk. Yet here was a culture that did not have the technology to pasteurise, depended heavily on raw dairy and showed nothing but excellent health.

Dr Price was particularly impressed with the Native American Indians and spent considerable time in his book describing these people and their health. The Native Americans were renowned for their great strength and were often used by the pioneer circus sideshows to impress and astound others with their athletic prowess. They were also known to be particularly tall, with several reports estimating the height of the frontier Native American males as reaching around 7 foot tall. Early travellers across America noted how the American Indians hunted their food. When they hunted deer they did not hide themselves hoping to catch the deer unawares. They would literally chase after the deer and had sufficient stamina to keep on its tracks, until the deer itself became worn out. Then the fatiguing deer became easy prey for the strong Native Americans. The early Native Americans literally had greater stamina than strong deer!

Nutrition's Playground

Not only were the Native Americans exceptionally strong, but they also had fantastic facial structure, virtually perfect teeth, and wide dental arches. Price noted in one particular group of Indians that he examined, totalling 87 different individuals containing 2464 teeth, that they only had 4 teeth that had ever been attacked by dental cavities. Ultimately they had fewer cavities than the exceptionally healthy Swiss! So what did they eat? The environment was completely different than the mountainous valleys in Switzerland. The Native Americans were nomadic and followed the animal herds, wherever they went. They ate meat in abundance, but specifically sought after, the organs of the animals. They instinctively knew that many of the nutrients were to be found here. They also hunted animals seeking out those that had greater fat stored on their bodies. If they managed to kill an animal that was particularly lean it was common practice to remove the organs and leave the meat. Often these organs meats, being considered sacred foods, were saved for particularly needful groups of people such as young children, pregnant and lactating mothers and the elderly members of the tribe. They were seen as people who required the greatest nutritional intake possible. They were often given preferential choice over these sacred foods.

I found it particularly inspiring to read about the South Sea Islanders. I'm sure this is because I lived in the Fiji Islands for six years as a teenager. Even after 75 years I was still able to see for myself some of the observations, habits and cultural foods that Price talked about, from his journey. Dr Price noted that most of the woman looked like sisters and the men looked like brothers. Now this was partly because they were a fairly closed population group and there was very similar genetics as they were on an isolated island. However, Price also put this down to the fact that the foods that people ate encouraged growth and development much closer to physical perfection. He was also aware of the great zest these people had for life. Even amongst the younger teenagers within the tribes Price found optimism, vitality and happiness amongst the South Sea Islanders. One of my long abiding memories of living in the Fiji islands is the broad, white teeth and smiles that were constantly upon the faces of the local Islanders. The tourism industry promotes these islands as one of the friendliest destinations you could ever visit.

This was a particularly interesting find for Dr Price as he had found a culture that had a greater reliance upon plant and vegetable matter than what he had seen amongst the Swiss or the American Indians. They ate plenty of fruits and included some vegetables, particularly the starchy root crop taro. This was usually prepared by a fermentation process that left it sitting for up to two weeks in the ground. This served to pre-digest the starchy crop making it easier to stomach and metabolise. Coconut and coconut oil was also a commonly eaten food, finding its way into many of their local dishes. He also observed like the previous cultures he had seen an abundance and variety animal foods. There was particularly a preference for seafood, such as fish, octopus and crab. It was common practice to eat the whole fish including the head and when they ate crab they literally ate the whole animal. They would eat all the meat, the eggs and they would even crush the shell and make into a paste and included it in other foods that they prepared. Pork and lard was also on the menu as there were wild pigs that they hunted on occasion roaming the Island.

It amazes me how cultures even years later still hold onto traditions and habits that have been developed by previous generations! I was fortunate enough to make friends with people who lived a life away from the two major Fijian cities. Although they had been influenced by the Western world and had electricity, lighting and television, they still very much got their food from the land and the sea around them. They kept some cows, pigs and chickens and would often go out on their small boat to fish. Fish doesn't come any fresher than that! It would be pulled out of ocean and within minutes be nicely cooked and ready to eat and, just like the observations of Dr. Price over 70 years earlier, they relished the fish heads and eyes. These good friends had excellent teeth, broad faces, a contagious optimism about life and a great sense of humour. Most of the years that I lived in South Pacific were spent within the city limits, and here the observations of health were very different to the more natural setting of village life. Dentistry even in the 1990s was very expensive in Fiji. This meant that when the people suffered from dental cavities, as was typical when western foods are introduced, they could not afford to have their teeth repaired. This meant that many local Fijians had either missing teeth or obvious signs of cavities. However, their facial structure, health and strength were still fairly good. It must be remembered that Price concluded that dental cavities were the initial sign of ill health and that other disease processes tended to follow the appearance of cavities. He also observed it took up to 3 or 4 generations of eating devitalised food for widespread ill health to descend on a population.

Genetic variety

It would be a crime to study the work of Dr Weston A Price without taking some time to look at the African people that he visited. These were a particularly interesting group of people. The reason for this was that within a very small area Dr Price found several groups of people which were genetically very similar, but lived different lifestyles and therefore relied upon different foods. The first group that Price studied were the Masai and Samburu tribes. They were

33

Nutrition's Playground

predominantly cattle herders and relied heavily upon the produce that these animals provided them, namely blood, milk, and meat. The second group studied in Africa were hunters and gatherers and were found to be eating a variety of animals that they hunted and captured and also some plant seeds and vegetable matter. They would typically seek out and hunt the animals that were the fattest in that particular season or time of year. This meant that the foods they ate varied throughout the year. The last group of people were the agriculturalists and they relied more heavily upon the foods that they grew particularly certain grains, fruits and vegetables. However, it should be noted that even these farming people tended to eat a certain amount of animal food. Although they didn't rear and eat meat they did rely heavily upon a variety of different insects that made up about 10% of their diet. Here in Africa Price discovered a very special situation. All three groups of people ate whole, untouched, unprocessed foods! It was observed that as the people ate more plant matter their health wasn't quite as good as those that relied more upon the animal produce. When carrying out his dental cavity searches Dr Price studied over 700 different individuals amongst the Masai and found absolutely no cavities! As he investigated the hunter-gatherers and the agriculturalists the number of cavities increased slightly in each group. Amongst the agriculturalists about 6% of the mouths investigated were found to contain cavities. This is still significantly less than what you would expect to find in the mouths from those on a Western diet. The Masai were very tall people reaching heights of up to 7 feet; however, they tended to be very lean as well. The hunter-gatherers were not as tall but appeared to have better muscle mass and strength. The agriculturalists were still healthy specimens but were not as healthy as the other two groups. The African region taught Price one of his most important lessons. Even when people of the same genetic stock ate whole and nourishing foods across a wide spectrum from mostly plant

34

foods to mostly animal foods a very good level of health could be obtained. However, he also noted that the tribe with the very best of health from the 3 groups ate a better mix of both plant foods and animal foods. Optimal health requires nutrients present in both types of food.

There are so many lessons to learn from the travels and investigations of Dr Weston A Price. To fully appreciate what he did I can only recommend his book, Nutrition and Physical Degeneration. It is very informative, though not a read for the faint hearted. To try and more fully understand the many findings that Dr Price discovered it seems appropriate to summarise in brief many of the things that he advised.

In every culture without exception when Western foods of commerce were introduced to the native people it was soon followed with an increase in the incidence of dental cavities.

When Western foods were eaten amongst native cultures, the next generation exhibited narrowed dental arches, narrower faces and less sturdy bone structure. It was also very common to find that there was a higher rate of ill health and disease amongst this new generation.

Despite the varied terrains, altitudes, environments, and foods available to these people it was clear that they had great knowledge of how to maximise the nutrients available to them in the foods that were present in their surroundings.

Each of the 15 traditional cultures that were visited ate animal produce as part of their regular diet.

Nutrition's Playground

Traditional populations ate four times the calcium and other minerals and at least ten times the fat soluble nutrients, vitamins A, D and K2, compared to western populations

Through the surveys and studies of these diets he prioritised the foods that were most commonly eaten. This is a prioritised list of these foods:

- Fish and shellfish were most commonly eaten, followed by birds including their organs and the skin of the birds.

- Red meats were often consumed along with the organs and especially the fat that was found on the carcass. In

- Many cases the fat was indeed the preferred nutrient and was intensely sought after!

- Raw dairy produce was an important part of some of the cultures, though not all had access to milk producing animals.

- Where available eggs were often eaten, followed by reptiles and insects in some of the more remote areas where many of the foods above were difficult to come across.

It is clear that animal life played a vital role in the health and physical superiority of many of the indigenous cultures from all over the globe. There was one objective that Dr Price had at the beginning of his travels that he was unable to realise. He had set out hoping to be able to find a culture that was living predominantly a vegetarian regime. He did not find this dietary approach in any area of the world that he travelled to. The answers to this conundrum were answered within the walls of his laboratory where he had sent many food samples whilst he was travelling the globe. He found that certain nutrients were only present in animal foods at the levels needed to generate full health. In particular Price identified a number of nutrients he referred to as the fat-soluble activators. Vitamins A and D have very specific purposes in the body and are involved in a vast myriad of chemical and cellular processes. A very specific factor associated with the health of all these cultures was something that Price referred to as activator X. This was a nutrient only found in foods from animals that grazed on fast growing green grass. Unfortunately in all the work Price did he was unable to document exactly what this X factor was. Although he was able to identify rich sources of activator X, such high vitamin butter oil. Since that time science has uncovered a new vitamin, called vitamin K2, which has continued to show many similarities with the observations Price made regarding activator X. Many believe that this nutrient is in fact the elusive activator X that Price so highly prized.

Modern Pioneers

In more recent years the Weston A Price foundation set up in 1999 by Sally Fallon, a wonderful nutrition pioneer herself, discovered many other reasons why each of these traditional cultures always had animal products in their diet. The foundation has particularly encouraged the intake of traditional fats because of these vital nutrients that are required in our diet. The other nutrients essential to health are cholesterol, despite current opinion on this nutrient, vitamin B12, and three specific super long chain saturated fatty acids; arachidonic acid (AA), eicosapentaenoic acid (EPA) and docosahexaenoic acid (DHA). EPA and DHA are

Nutrition's Playground

more commonly known today as the omega-3 fats. They've received a lot of press attention in recent years and we now find many food products claiming to have added Omega 3 for our nutritional benefit. The Weston A Price foundation along with Dr Price himself currently recognizes that there are certain nutrients that are often present in plants but are much more easily absorbed from animal produce. These nutrients are essential to good health and well-being. They include calcium, vitamins B6, magnesium, iron, zinc and copper. Now it would be foolish at this point to say that we do not get many of these nutrients in our current diet! Obviously these nutrients are present in foods despite the level of processing and manufacturing we put foods through. Perhaps Price's biggest finding was the fact that the civilised diet of his day, the 1930s, had significantly lower nutrient intakes than one the primitive indigenous cultures that he studied. His research discovered that the primitive diets contained 4 times the amount of calcium and other minerals and as much as 10 times the level of fat-soluble activators like vitamin A, vitamin D and activator X (vitamin K2) than the typical American diet of his day! This was because traditional wisdom had come to treasure a variety of foods across the generations that had become so important to their health that they referred to them as 'sacred' foods. Price discovered that it was these sacred foods that ensured health and vitality from generation to generation because they were so rich in the fat soluble activators and key minerals. Traditional diets emphasised organ meats over muscle meats, animal fats, raw or fermented dairy products, fish and shellfish, fermented vegetables, soaked or fermented grains, bone broths and other nutrient dense, naturally occurring foods. In today's world we can only assume with the vast increase in processing over the last 30 years that the nutrient value of food has only got worse. This distinct lack of micronutrients is one of the reasons why we see so much illness in the

Nutrition's Playground

Western world despite vast amounts of money being invested in medication and modern science.

It boggles the mind to think that Dr Price did all of this research over 70 to 80 years ago and yet today it still has immense value and increases our understanding of the nutritional requirements of the human body. Our nutrient requirements in this stressful and very busy world are probably greater than they were back in the 1930s. So the need to locate and include nutrient dense food in our everyday diet is higher than ever before. The pivotal role that Dr Price played cannot be underestimated!

Nutrition's Playground

Step 3: Widespread Whitewash

Processing food brings about ill health! This is undoubtedly one of the key facts Weston A Price identified as he travelled around the globe studying the eating habits of traditional cultures. When these primitive cultures were exposed to Western trading and commerce, often through trading ports by rivers or seas, a disturbing change in their health began to occur without exception. The very first observation was a huge increase in the number of dental cavities. This often lead over time to a continued depreciation in health and the occurrence of disease previously unheard of amongst these indigenous people. Even more fascinating than that was the observations Price made in the next-generation. Where parents had consumed Western foods their offspring had noticeably narrower dental arches and reduced immunity, which caused them to suffer from the same illnesses that one would have expected in Western society at that time. They seemed to lose the vigour and vitality he had seen in so many of these traditional cultures around the world.

This was exactly what Dr Price had been looking for! He had been seeking to know what caused so many dental cavities in mainstream civilised people. He had observed healthy cultures with virtually no dental cavities or disease and he had observed the same genetic stock go on to develop cavities and the same diseases observed in Western cultures. This

Nutrition's Playground

enabled Price to make a more detailed study of the different nutrition between these groups of people. This proved to be a master stroke of genius! This is how Price was able to identify the distinct lack of micronutrients in the modern diet. Dr Price also singled out specific foods that seemed to be causing many of the problems he had observed. These four foods known by some health experts as the four white devils, are refined white flour, pasteurised milk, refined white sugar and processed table salt. In this chapter we are going to investigate what it is about these four foods that wreak havoc with our bodies!

White Flour

Wheat has been a staple in our society now for literally thousands of years. Research has identified evidence of harvested grains of wild einkorn, an early ancestor to wheat, as far back as 16,000 BC. There is evidence of many other types of grain being grown and eaten since that time, including varieties such as triticum, emmer and spelt. However, the flour that we eat in society today is far removed from the nurturing food that supported generations in years gone by. These differences start with the species of wheat grown on mass, a genetically altered hybrid of wheat produced to meet commercial needs. The harsh milling methods, the chemicals added, and the many additional ingredients added to wheat-based foods, like bread, also contributes to the problem.

Common bread flour, milled from triticum aestivum, has the same ancestry as spelt, but exhibits the beneficial characteristic of grain kernels that thresh free of their hulls. This is clearly a time saver, as it eliminates the lengthy process of rubbing the grains free from their hulls. Worldwide wheat production in 2004 was approximately 624

41

million tonnes of wheat. The huge popularity of this grain is much more recent than perhaps many would realise.

Historical grains

In the early 1700s rye was a very popular grain amongst Europeans compromising as much as 40% of all their breads. However, by the early 1800s that percentage was down to barely 5%. In Scotland it was very rare to find anybody eating wheat bread as part of their diet except the very wealthy. By the 1850s all classes, including the working and labouring classes, ate wheat bread regularly. By 1860 the Americans were exporting vast amounts of wheat across the sea to Europe to try and meet demand. From a rarely used grain, we see within the short space of a hundred years wheat became the number one grain product used throughout the Western world.

With the advent of the industrial age Great Britain and America, who were to become some of the wealthiest nations, soon developed a reputation for producing some of the worst bread. This is probably in part down to the fact that industrialisation sought to produce large amounts of bread by mechanical means, and so the artisan baker became a much rarer breed. In 1771 Tobias Smollett wrote

'The bread I eat in London is a deleterious paste, mixed up with chalk, alum and bone ashes, insipid to the taste and destructive to the constitution.'

It wasn't that uncommon to find heavy metals being used in bread making during this period of time. During the 19th century both the US and UK finally passed laws criminalising food adulteration to stop some of the worst abuses of heavy metals being used in food. This prevented the modernised

Nutrition's Playground

bread making industry using aluminium sulphate to whiten their bread since its multiple poisoning effects are clearly understood in scientific literature.

If we jump forward to more modern history, we find that in 1910 about 70% of all American households baked their own bread at home. Something significant must have changed during the First World War because by 1924 only 30% of people baked their own bread at home! It was shortly after this that governments decided to begin enriching bread with synthetic vitamins and minerals as a way of trying to prevent deficiency and illness. It is interesting to note how much nutrition-oriented research followed immediately after both the First and Second World War. From the First World War onwards the baking industries continued to find smoother and better ways to produce the ultimate loaf. As business empires grew projected profit margins and the 'bottom line' soon became the motivation behind bread production. The mechanisation of production lines was all about producing a uniform loaf of bread at higher speed.

In 1961 the Chorleywood bread process was born. This method depends on high-speed mixers, chemical oxidants, solid vegetable fats, commercial yeast and water, followed by a complex mechanical process to produce a uniform loaf of bread sliced and packaged within 3 ½ hours. From this time onwards the days of taking time to prove, rise and allow bread to ferment to bring out the full flavour were long gone. The Chorleywood bread process revolutionised the industry and has become the norm in many countries around the world for mass-produced bread. Scientists have since produced hybrid forms of wheat with higher protein content so that these grains can cope with the larger amounts of abuse received through this mechanised process. The thought process is astounding! Rather than find appropriate ways to produce good bread with natural occurring wheat, they first mechanised the process, increased the speed of production and then developed a hybrid version of wheat that is more suited to the process that has been devised! Is it the horse or cart that is meant to go first?

Modern milling

With some of these historical facts still ringing in your mind, let's turn our attention to the modern day milling process that takes place before we even begin to utilise it in food. Towards the end of the 19th century a new method of grinding wheat was developed. This completely changed the rate and ability to grind large amounts of flour at a time. It was called the steel roller mill and was invented by a Swiss man named Helfenburger. This method of milling crushes the grains between a series of metal rollers. After each set of rollers has crushed the grain any fine flour particles are sifted out whilst the remaining partially compacted grains move on to the next set of rollers for further milling. Ironically today when you buy wholemeal flour, it has gone through the roller milling process to become pure white flour, then the bran and fibre sifted out during processing is added back into the flour in controlled measures! So, after all that, you might not even be getting the whole grain, perhaps only part of the fibre and bran that was originally contained within the grain. This system has enabled grain to be milled at much higher speeds, which inevitably has led to an increase in temperature experienced between each set of metal rollers. The higher temperature has a negative effect upon the grain.

Let's take a moment to consider the humble grain of wheat. The purpose of the grain of wheat, apart from being a food and energy store, is for the growth and continuation of the species. If a grain of wheat falls to the ground but the

Nutrition's Playground

conditions are not ideal for growth, it is able to lay dormant for many years until the conditions change to those that are more appropriate. Each grain has been designed and constructed carefully by nature to protect its vital contents. The outer layer or husk is a strong insoluble coating and keeps the elements out and the nutrients in. Contained inside the husk are three distinct parts, the bran, the germ, and the endosperm. The endosperm is basically a cell of energy to help fuel the early growth of the plant until it shoots forth leaves to enable it to generate energy through photosynthesis. The germ and the bran contain key nutrients and vital genetic information needed for the growth of the plant. Inside the grain there are also a number of powerful anti-nutrients. Phytic acid, an organic acid in which phosphorus is bound, enzyme inhibitors, tannins, complex sugars, gluten and other hard to digest proteins are all contained within the grain to preserve its valuable inner contents and prevent sprouting until the conditions are just right. Plants, grains included, need moisture, warmth, time and slight acidity in order to sprout. As the grain begins to sprout the phytic acid and enzyme inhibitors are neutralised, the tannins, complex sugars, gluten and other hardy substances are partially broken down into simpler components. Basically the plant's preservation methods are systematically removed allowing the plants to flourish and grow.

The need for speed and increased profit means that grains are thrown through the roller mill with no prior preparation. First and foremost this means that all of those preservative compounds that prevent the grain from sprouting are still contained within the end product, the flour. Is this a problem? Indeed it is! Phytic acid has the ability to bind to other minerals in the gut, like calcium, magnesium, copper, iron and especially zinc which then prevents their absorption into the blood. Inside the grain it is necessary to hold on to and protect these minerals from oxidation in preparation for the growth of the plant. In the gut this can prove problematic as it may lead to mineral deficiencies and potential bone deterioration as a result of lacking calcium and phosphorus. The enzyme inhibitors, tannins, sugars and proteins within the grain help to preserve, but in the gut they can become highly irritating and may cause allergies, digestive disorders and inflammation. So even if all we did was mill the grains of wheat and eat them we would still be likely to react negatively to this food. After all, we are eating the preservative, mineral blocking compounds that are naturally contained within the grain. Unfortunately we are not just eating ground up wheat! There is yet more to this story that needs to be told.

The steel rollers within the mill spin at great speeds generating huge amounts of friction and high temperatures. The increased temperatures play havoc with the delicate nutrients contained within the grain. Proteins become denatured, the fragile mono and polyunsaturated fats become oxidised and rancid and many of the vitamins are destroyed, especially vitamin E. The milling process sifts out the bran and germ leaving behind the fine particles of the endosperm. Remember, many of the nutrients are contained within the germ. With that sifting process we can say goodbye to much of the nutrition that was contained within. The flour at this point looks like a dirty, off-white powder. Most commercial mills bleach their flour to make it appear even more white, thus indicating a pure product. One of the most common substances used to bleach flour is benzoyl peroxide, which is the active ingredient in many acne creams and hair dyes. Another common bleaching agent is chlorine dioxide, a potent poison also used to bleach paper products and textiles. Which would you prefer, off-white flour or a potent bleaching agent that will irritate your gut and have toxic effects?

Nutrition's Playground

Simply intolerant

The ability to produce fine flour has become so advanced that the particles are like dust. Scientists have identified a condition called leaky gut syndrome that is aggravated by this extra fine flour. Leaky gut is evidenced by inflammation of the gut wall. The swelling of the cells leads to 'gaps' in the tight junctions between the gut and the blood stream. The fine flour particles may pass or 'leak' through the intestine wall into the blood stream without being fully digested. This is not normal and so a compound that should not be in the blood has now entered and is seen by the body as a foreign invader. The body immediately sets off a chain reaction and white blood cells respond as the immune system tries to protect the body from this unfamiliar compound. The more often this occurs the stronger the body's immune response becomes as the natural antibodies learn to recognise the 'invader' more quickly. The immune system soon uses the markers within the wheat as a stimulus for a response. Consequently if any wheat is eaten at all, even if fully digested, it sets off an inflammatory immune response. This may be what many people experience as gluten intolerance or inflammatory bowel syndrome (IBS). So the real question here is, Does gluten intolerance and the inability to properly break down and absorb certain grains come about as a result of fate, weak digestion or is it because the grains and the way they are processed make them indigestible? I would bank on the latter. Grains have successfully been the 'staff of life' for generations, without the growing problems of intolerance we are experiencing in modern times.

The extra fine white flour that is universally sought after, even when it is tolerated without an inflammatory response, still instigates problems within the body. The flour particles have about 10,000 times the surface area of a single grain of wheat, allowing the digestive enzymes of the gut to work exceptionally quickly in breaking down the polysaccharides, or complex sugars, into simple sugars like glucose for absorption into the blood. This ultimately increases blood sugar levels at a phenomenal rate! Refined white breads, like baguettes, have the ability to increase blood sugars almost as quickly as pure glucose, which requires no digestion in the gut and can be absorbed immediately. High blood sugars need to be tempered by the pancreas, which sends out a hormone called insulin to facilitate the passage of sugars into the cells of the body, lowering total blood sugar. High blood insulin levels are associated with energy storage. When insulin levels are high, fat burning is suppressed and fat storage is increased. This means that regular intake of cheap, refined white bread; pasta or flour products can be easily converted and assist in the storage of body fat! But this also increases the demand on the pancreas to produce insulin to control excess blood sugar and is almost certainly a contributing factor in the development of diabetes. To make matters worse most refined white flour is deficient in necessary vitamins and minerals as a result of the harsh milling process. This means that the body has no choice but to utilise its own limited store of micronutrients to actually digest and metabolise the flour. The net consequence is a decrease in vitamins and minerals within the body!

Grains have been a staple in many populations for thousands of years. They are a nutritious food and should be consumed as part of a healthy diet. However, there is no way our major source of grain, refined white flour, can be placed under the heading 'nutritious'.

Nutrition's Playground

Pasteurised Milk

Kurt Oster, Chief of Cardiology and chairman of the Department of Medicine at Park City hospital in Bridgeport, Connecticut, with over 20 years of experience in this role made this comment:

'Milk has changed over the years by processing into an unrecognisable physicochemical emulsion, which bears very little resemblance to the original, natural, and nutritional milk.'

How many years does it take for us to consider somebody an expert? Is 50 years of faithful devotion to a single industry sufficient? Dan Logue is a dairy farmer with exactly those credentials who remarked about modern milk:

'Pasteurised, homogenised milk? Might as well drink water with chalk in it.'

Both of these comments, from highly respected experts in their field, should help to stimulate a few probing questions about the quality of the milk we are drinking today. Those who have been around for more than a quarter of a century will likely remember the days when the local milkman delivered milk to the door. Milk used to come in glass bottles, not plastic or cardboard containers. Almost always you were able to see the cream separated from the liquid sitting on the surface. Any delay in collecting your milk from the front doorstep would often result in finding a nice hole in the top of the tinfoil lid. The local birds certainly appreciated the cream that had settled on the surface of the milk. Perhaps they knew something instinctively that we have failed to recognize for many years. The milk processors of modern day have saved us the hassle of leaving a pint of milk out to have the cream removed by the birds. We can purchase milk with all the cream already removed. Oh, the convenience of skimmed milk!

Dairy-licious

To more fully understand what Dr Oster was talking about when he said that milk today is vastly different from the original product, we need to take some time to understand what happens to raw milk once it reaches the dairy. It is very difficult today for a regular person to receive access or to visit a modern dairy processing plant. Safety and hygiene are of the utmost importance, so visitors are kept to virtually zero. Emily Green, a journalist, provided a rare glimpse into the workings of a modern-day dairy when she wrote in the Los Angeles Times:

'Inside the plant, all you can see is stainless steel. Inside that machinery, milk shipped from the farm is remade. First it is separated in centrifuges into fat, protein and various other solids and liquids. Once segregated, these are reconstituted to set levels for whole, low-fat and non-fat milk. What is left over will go to butter, cream, cheese, dried milk and a host of other milk products. Of the reconstituted milks, whole milk will most closely approximate original cow's milk. When fat is removed, it is replaced with protein and vitamin rich skimmed milk powder or concentrate. Standardisation ensures that milk is consistent, that one glass of any given type tastes exactly like the next.

Then milk is pasteurised at 161 degrees (Fahrenheit) for 15 seconds by rushing the milk past superheated stainless steel plates. If the temperature is 200, it is called Ultra pasteurised. This will have a distinct cooked milk taste but it is sterile and can be sold on grocery shelves. It does not even require refrigeration... once processed, the milk will last for weeks not days.'

Nutrition's Playground

It is astounding to think that even whole milk is completely separated in to its component parts before it is reconstituted as pseudo whole milk! Can it be right that modern dairies disintegrate nature's perfect food and then rebuild it, but in doing so set their own parameters as to how much fat and protein should be contained within it? Raw milk from Friesian or Holstein cows, the most common milk producing variety, typically contains 3.4 - 3.9% fat, but following a trip to the dairy 'whole' milk is standardised at 3.25-3.5% fat. Semi skimmed milk is standardised at between 1.5 - 1.8% fat, whilst skimmed milk contains only 0.1% fat. This is very beneficial to the dairy because every variety removes some of the butterfat. They can make much more money selling the butterfat as cream, ice cream or butter than they can by selling it as milk. However, a problem is created when they remove the butterfat. The milk loses its texture and body, so all reduced fat milks have dried skimmed milk powder added to them to 'correct' this problem. This added ingredient will not be identified on the label as it is considered a part of the original product. This is misleading because semi skimmed and skimmed milk has been changed into an unnaturally high protein, low fat product. This makes the milk deficient or devoid in fat-soluble vitamin A, a necessary nutrient for the assimilation of proteins.

It is important to make a little side note on how skimmed milk powder is produced. Complex machinery is used to force milk through a tiny hole at very high pressure after which it is blown out into a high temperature spray drier. Not only does this cause the milk to become powder very quickly, but also the natural cholesterol that is contained within the milk becomes oxidised. At a future point in this book I will discuss fats and cholesterol, but at this point it is valuable to know that cholesterol is essential to our health. We shouldn't be worried about cholesterol in our food.

Nutrition's Playground

However, we do not want to be eating oxidised cholesterol! Oxidised cholesterol has been implicated in feeding the build-up of plaque in our arteries, a condition that the medical establishment refers to as atherosclerosis. We've been told time and time again that too much fat in our diet will contribute to heart disease. So when the health-conscious customer purchases semi-skimmed or skimmed milk in an attempt to lower their fat intake and therefore be heart friendly, they are consuming oxidised cholesterol from the added milk powder, which will ironically contribute to the process of heart disease.

It would be wise at this point to summarise the negative nutritional side effects of pasteurisation upon milk.

Pasteurised milk contains less than 10% of the original enzymes.

Proteins are denatured by the heat, particularly lysine and tyrosine, resulting in serious loss of metabolic availability.

Of the 18 fatty acids present in milk many will have been altered by the heat, especially the 10 essential unsaturated fats.

The loss of fat-soluble vitamins A, D, E and K could run as high as 66%. Vitamin C loss usually exceeds 50%, whilst losses of other water-soluble vitamin losses often run from 38 to 80%.

The most common sugar in milk, lactose, becomes less metabolically available because the enzyme lactase needed for its absorption has been destroyed during pasteurisation.

Nutrition's Playground

Calcium is altered by heat becoming insoluble and loss of metabolism may run 50% or more.

The loss of virtually all friendly lactic acid bacteria may leave surviving pathogenic bacteria freedom to multiply.

Milky Marketing

Milk is a natural emulsion; when shaken the fat globules disperse throughout; if it is allowed to stand the cream of natural milk will float to the top because it is less dense than the rest of the fluid. In times past the consumer had always used the cream line and colour as an indicator of the quality of the milk. A larger volume of cream and a subtle yellow colour were markers that indicated better quality. Pasteurisation of milk enabled the dairy processors to transport milk over large distances without the milk souring or going bad. They soon realised during long journeys that the milk separated into liquid and cream, which began to pose problems in emptying their tankers upon delivery.

The process of homogenisation was originally devised in 1899 as an answer to this problem. Homogenisation is the process of forcing milk through hair like tubes at extremely high pressure, around 2100 psi. This breaks down the fat globules into microscopic, irrecoverable particles that will never combine back together and settle on the surface of the milk. Modern dairies pass milk through two separate homogenising valves to be sure the process is carried out effectively. This mechanised process certainly solved the problem of transportation, but for over 30 years the general public opinion was not positive towards homogenised milk. For a start it had changed the taste, and also they no longer had a method of determining the quality of the milk because the cream never settled on the surface to reveal the volume or colour of the cream! This has since enabled lower quality milk to be produced and sold as all milk is now standardised to look and taste the same.

Earlier it was noted that modern society is experiencing a growing amount of intolerance to wheat as a result of 'leaky gut' and a degree of indigestibility experienced with rapidly milled flour. A similar story is found with the use of modern pasteurised milk. The number of people reporting allergies to dairy foods, or lactose intolerance, seems also to be increasing year by year. There are many popular arguments that have been postulated to explain the adverse affects of milk on some individuals. A quick search on the internet reveals claims of anywhere from 25 – 70% of the global population are already lactose intolerant because it is not a part of their genetic make up, neither was it a part of their traditional food culture. Others argue that we are indeed the only species to drink the milk of another species of animal and therefore it is logical that we should not be drinking cow's milk because no other animal would do that. These arguments are weak at best.

Milked up charges

In order to know that as much as 70% of the population were intolerant would require a study of considerable magnitude and funding. A significant sample of every culture of every country around the world would need to be surveyed and tested for their ability to tolerate dairy foods and, at best, have a lactose reaction test performed! No study to date has been performed in this manner, suggesting that these figures are extrapolated from small-scale research and then estimated across the globe. For example official statistics from the National Institute of Diabetes, Digestive and Kidney Disorders (NIDDK) on the topic of lactose intolerance have been drawn from a simple, self-reported census. How reliable

Nutrition's Playground

can self-reported statistics be in relation to national or global data? Another set of global figures published several years ago in Scientific American, tested a variety of population groups including 20 subjects amongst American Blacks and 315 subjects for American Caucasians. This is hardly accurate and wide reaching enough to begin suggesting that nearly 1 in 2 should avoid milk. It seems illogical to suggest that because no other animal species drinks another species milk that we are somewhat unusual because we do. No other species mass-produces grains, vegetables, fruit, eggs or meat either! Does that mean we should stop eating these too because we are unique in the animal world? We eat the meat of other animals just like other animal species – so their cells, tissues and nutritive components are ending up inside us for digestion and assimilation. This is the same for many species of animal. What difference does it make if it is meat or milk? It comes from the same source! Animals act by instinct and would clearly not allow another animal to enjoy their milk because protective mechanisms within would fight back out of fear.

Humans are blessed with greater intellect and, sitting at the top of the food chain, so to speak, have domesticated the cow and have that to our advantage. We can use their milk and benefit from it. It should also be noted that nearly every culture around the world follows natural instinct to breastfeed children. Human breast milk is somewhat different in nutrient composition to cow's milk. The main difference is it is much sweeter. See the comparison below:

- Human milk by weight contains, on average, 1.1% protein, 4.2% fat, 7.0% lactose, and supplies 72 kcal of energy per 100 grams

Nutrition's Playground

- Cow's milk by weight contains, on average, 3.4% protein, 3.6% fat, and 4.6% lactose, and supplies 66 kcal of energy per 100 grams

It is clear that human milk has much higher sugar content with 7% lactose as well as a higher fat content. Breast milk is without question the best food source for any child, providing the mother is healthy. This would logically suggest to me that every individual who was ever breastfed was able to fully digest and assimilate lactose in considerable amounts during the early years of their life. Why then are we seeing so much intolerance, specifically to lactose, in Western culture? Just like flour and gluten intolerance it's not just the body reacting to an inability to digest the milk, but that the milk has been rendered indigestible because of the processes of pasteurisation and homogenisation.

It was stated earlier that pasteurisation destroys over 90% of all enzymes in milk. In some dairies the test to check that pasteurisation has been successful is to test for the presence of enzymes. The milk is passed when no enzymes are present. This means that the enzyme lactase, needed by the body to digest and absorb lactose in milk, has also been destroyed. Without the lactase it is unrealistic to expect the body to be able to break down the lactose sugar; it's impossible without the natural catalyst. The body may begin to react to this indigestible sugar if it cannot produce sufficient lactase from within and as a result lactose intolerance and its frustrating symptoms become apparent. Lactose intolerance therefore is not an allergic reaction, but an enzyme deficiency that is perhaps caused and certainly aggravated by pasteurisation.

In a similar way that the milling of wheat and grains creates devitalised food, it is difficult to see how the rigorous and

56

damaging processes of pasteurising, homogenising and skimming milk would result in a nutritious food

White Refined Sugar

Sugar has been a part of recorded human dietary consumption since around 510 BC. Emperor Darius of Persia invaded India and found the 'reed that gives honey without bees', a fairly accurate description of sugar cane. Sugar cane was held for many years under great secrecy whilst being exported for a rich profit. In the 7th century AD, as a result of the expansion of the Arab peoples, sugar cane was discovered during their invasion of Persia. They took this new plant and carried it with them for production in other regions that they conquered. Sugar was discovered by western Europeans as a result of the crusades in the 11th century. The first recorded use of sugar in England was in 1099. During the centuries to follow trade between the east and west increased, in which sugar played an increasingly important role. It was a luxury item that sold at a high price.

Shortly after the Americas were discovered it is recorded that sugar cane was taken to the Caribbean in 1493 where, because of the warm, humid climate, it grew extremely well. On the back of the slave trade plantations the sugar industry was quickly established in that region. By 1750 there were 120 sugar refineries operating in Britain turning out a combined output of 30,000 tons of sugar. Sugar was still a luxury item and was making vast profits, so the government taxed it heavily. In 1815 the British government gathered a staggering £3 million in sugar taxes! In 1874 a key event in the history of sugar occurred when Prime Minister Gladstone abolished the tax and brought the price of sugar within reach of the ordinary citizens. Since that time sugar production and consumption has risen steadily.

Nutrition's Playground

Sugar is now produced in over 121 countries with global production in excess of 140 million tons in 2004. The European Union, Brazil and India are the top three producers accounting for 40% of annual global production. The climate greatly determines what crop is used in sugar production. Warmer climates account for 70% of sugar production through sugar cane farming, whereas the remaining 30% comes from more temperate climates using sugar beets.

Health sweet

There is no doubt that we live in a world that is driven by our sweet taste buds! The Western world has become addicted to sugar and calorific sugar alternatives in a way that can only lead to disaster. Bill Misner PhD says:

'The health dangers ingested sugar creates when habitually imposed upon human physiology are certain. Simple sugars have been observed to aggravate asthma, muster mental illness, move mood swings, provoke personality changes, nourish nervous disorders, hurry heart disease, deliver diabetes, grow gallstones, hasten hypertension, add arthritis, and on top of all of that...It will kill you!'

Eating three quarters of your own body weight in sugar, syrups and refined sweeteners each year, combined with the negative side effects of such compounds, does not generate thoughts of a positive future for those of us who live in Western civilisation! But, as just stated, it wasn't always like that. Sugar consumption in such large amounts has only been a factor of the last 100 years or so since the British government stopped taxing it and made it affordable to the masses. Sugar is no longer seen as the must-have luxury item it once was, but as a common place food stuff found in every home bringing with it dental decay, disrupted blood sugar,

Nutrition's Playground

mood swings, hormonal imbalance, weak bones and the not-so slow road to obesity.

Do we know that sugar is harmful to our health? Are the dangers of sugar still hidden from us? I think the answer to both questions, unfortunately, may still be yes! The message of the dangers of sugar has permeated society and many health-conscious shoppers take care and strive to avoid the glut of sugar currently available to us. But yet, somehow, it continues to sneak into our diets under our very noses.

In 2002 it was reported in the Guardian newspaper that sugar consumption in the UK had increased to 30kg per person per year. The total intake of all calorific sugars and syrups in England in 2002 was determined by the British Heart Foundation to be 49kg per person per year! In the USA sugar consumption actually declined between 1974 and 1986 as many sweetened beverages replaced sugar with High fructose corn syrup (HFCS). However, the total amount of calorific sweeteners has increased and was reported to be a total of 69kg per person per year in 1996! Manufacturers and food companies are clearly succeeding in pulling the wool over the eyes of the general public. They are able to report that actual sugar consumption has decreased and to identify less added sugar on the labels of their food products. This is obviously the wolf in sheep's clothing as they continue to boost the calorific content of their products by adding in highly refined alternatives from other sources like corn syrups and fruit concentrates.

Nearly 60% of all sugar ingested by the average Westerner is taken in as an ingredient hidden within processed foods. The list of refined sugar alternatives is quite substantial and includes products, such as:

Nutrition's Playground

- Dextrose

- Maltodextrin

- Inverted sugar syrup

- Glucose-Fructose syrup

- High Fructose corn syrup

- Fructose

- Sorbitol

- Mannitol

- Xylitol

- Fruit concentrate

Most of these ingredients carry the same amount of calories as sugar, chemically known as sucrose, at 4 calories per gram. But often the general public either does not look at the ingredients list, or are unaware of the terminology to know that they are still eating a product that contains a high proportion of refined sugars. The front of the food package may also indicate that the food has no added sugar, because technically refined, white sugar has not been added, but perhaps sorbitol or fructose has! Manufacturers may rely on public ignorance or indifference when using sugars like fructose. They are happy to inform people that fructose is derived from fruit and therefore a healthy sugar. Why should that make any difference? White, refined sugar is derived from plants too, cane and beets! Fructose is also a highly processed sugar. It does not naturally exist on its own as a sugar. In most fruit fructose is usually combined in a 50/50 split with glucose. Some fruits, like apples, pears and grapes have a naturally higher fructose level compared to glucose, but these are the exceptions rather than the rule. This is often why the sweet fruit concentrate added as an apparently 'healthy' alternative is usually derived from these three fruits. Fructose is sweeter than sucrose and as such smaller amounts can be used to impart the same sweetness. In order to produce high fructose syrups or pure fructose, the glucose needs to be removed or converted. This is most commonly done by enzymatically changing glucose to fructose in controlled levels.

Fructose frustration

Studies on fructose as a pure sugar or high fructose concentrated syrups have demonstrated detrimental side effects to human health. Pure fructose, just like pure sugar contains no minerals or enzymes to help digest or assimilate it into the body. This means that it robs the body of vital micronutrient stores in the process of metabolism. These vitamins and minerals are necessary for long term health. We must make deposits of these nutrients often in our diet. If too many withdrawals are made, as occurs when refined sugars, like sucrose and fructose, are eaten the nutrient account will soon become overdrawn. This is when we will notice the negative side effects on our health as the early signs of chronic illness begin to set in. Micronutrient bankruptcy is something that everyone should be seeking to avoid. Studies have shown that fructose increases our losses of both calcium and phosphorus. Fructose has also been shown to interfere with the heart's use of key minerals like magnesium, copper and chromium. It has been implicated in blood clotting and inhibiting the immune response of white blood cells. Also

Nutrition's Playground

because fructose is metabolised completely by the liver it does not stimulate insulin from the pancreas the way sugar does. Fructose is converted to fat and cholesterol that are retained in the blood more effectively than any other sugar. Since the introduction of fructose and high fructose syrups the rate of obesity in the USA and the UK has risen considerably and is certainly one of the many contributing factors to the growing dilemma. But still the food processors set about generating a positive profile for fruit-based, 'healthy' fructose! Perhaps the biggest reason for a shift to fructose is that it is 70% sweeter than sucrose and so smaller amounts may be used to achieve the same sweetness and therefore increase profit margins.

The sugar industry has been a profit making giant for several generations and it is not likely to just sit back and whimper into submission. We can see that despite the growing caution that the public have developed towards sugar, it has barely made a dent in business figures. The industry has remained one step ahead by including sugars in readymade processed foods, which the public are less likely to source out, and by using alternative sources of sugar that the public are less familiar with, even marketing some as 'better' for us!

Processed Table Salt

Salt has been a part of the human food supply for literally thousands of years. It has been sought after, harvested and traded throughout the generations as a medicinal nutrient and a key to health. There are many recorded references to salt. The earliest known reference from the Chinese Peng Tzao-Kan-Mu is dated at 2700 B.C. It delicately describes over 40 kinds of salt and some methods of extraction. The Bible contains many interesting references to salt. Matthew 5:13 provides an invaluable insight:

Nutrition's Playground

'Ye are the salt of the earth: but if the salt have lost his savour,
wherewith shall it be salted? It is thenceforth good for nothing, but
to be cast out, and to be trodden under foot of men.'

Although Jesus Christ was sharing significant, spiritual
teachings in his famous 'sermon on the mount', this particular
point was a comparison that the people of the day knew and
understood only too well. That is, salt from the earth is
invaluable to add flavour and nutrient value to a meal.
However, the people knew well that if the salt had become
contaminated so as to 'lose its savour', it no longer was able
to provide those same nutritive and taste-enhancing benefits.
Salt does not go bad, rancid or degrade. The only way salt
would lose its savour was for it to become mixed with some
other compound that corrupted its purity, rendering it
undesirable. Why compare people to salt? In the meridian of
time salt was highly prized and understood for its nutritive
and life-giving properties. Christ was placing a high value on
the people he was addressing by comparing them to pure salt.

Ready Salted

In modern day the value on salt has completely changed. It is
still a significant trading commodity. World salt production
in 2006 was estimated to be over 240 million tons, with China
and the USA producing almost half the total between them.
The UK produces approximately 5.8 million tons of salt. The
profitable value has changed, not because we don't use or
require salt, but as a simple rule of supply and demand.
There are such vast levels of salt production that salt between
2007 and early 2008 was traded on the stock market from 85p
to £1 per kilogram. Hardly the 'white gold' it once was.
Despite its lack lustre price tag, salt is still very much in
demand. Another question does need to be asked though. Is
the salt being traded today the same as the salt that Jesus
placed such a high value on?

Nutrition's Playground

There is another point worth considering first. Salt was highly prized during Biblical times and is documented throughout history as being valuable to many populations for its health promoting and medicinal purposes. However, it seems today no matter where you go there is a general consensus that salt is bad for health and is a significant contributor to elevated blood pressure and therefore heart disease. The US Food and Drug Administration and the UK Food Standards Agency both advocate limiting salt to no more than 6g per day with the intention that they will in time reduce this level further to between 1.5 – 3 g per day. They also identify that the majority of the general public in both countries eat much more than this as a result of eating processed and readymade foods. There have been numerous recent advertising campaigns and marketing changes to food products to teach the public about this need to lower salt intake. What has happened that has caused us to turn our backs on what was once considered so beneficial to our health? Surely we cannot be talking about the same basic mineral compound?

With such strong campaigns shouting about the dangers of excess salt in the diet it is only natural to assume that there must be a significant amount of research supporting such a claim. Perhaps because the guidance has been so strong we have assumed this is so obviously correct without feeling a need to look any deeper. It doesn't take too much digging to discover that this infallible evidence has a little more than a few cracks in it. A study published in the Journal of the American Medical Association (JAMA) in May 1998 reviewed 58 scientific trials dealing with hypertensive individuals and a further 56 trials investigating individuals with normal blood pressure. In conclusion it was stated:

*'A mean daily sodium reduction of 160 mmol/24 h for 7 days decreases BP by 1.2/0.3 mmHg in normotensive persons. **This effect size does not justify a general recommendation for***

64

Nutrition's Playground

reduced sodium intake (my emphasis). A mean daily sodium reduction of 118 mmol/24 h for 28 days decreases BP by 3.9/1.9 mmHg in hypertensive persons. This effect indicates that reduced sodium intake may be used as a supplementary treatment in hypertension.'

The effect of reducing salt across all the studies involved in the meta-analysis on people with normal blood pressure had so little an effect that it clearly does not support the recommendation to encourage the general populous to reduce salt. Salt reduction even for those with high blood pressure still only had minor effects and therefore only serves as a possible complement to other medications or therapies to lower blood pressure. These University of Copenhagen researchers reviewed 114 randomly chosen studies. Astonishingly they concluded that 'the benefit for hypertensives was significantly smaller than could be achieved by antihypertensive drugs' and that for normal individuals to reduce blood pressure by 'even a single millimetre of mercury could only be achieved with an extreme reduction in salt intake.' After publication in the Journal of the American Medical Association (JAMA), Drummond Rennie, the editor, said:

'The commitment to salt education goes way beyond scientific facts.'

The physician Lewis Dahl has often been cited as providing compelling evidence of the link between salt and increases in blood pressure. However, in 1979, a few years after his death, it was pointed out that the levels of salt he fed the rats in his study were equivalent to more than 500g a day for an adult human. This is highly unlikely to ever occur as levels of 20g a day are some of the highest recorded in population studies on human beings. Such extreme over feeding is not helpful in the search for the truth about salt as it is completely outside the frame of relevance. The Scottish Heart Health Study launched

65

Nutrition's Playground

in 1984 involved 7300 men, one of the largest intrapopulation groups ever studied on salt intakes. The British Medical Journal published the results 4 years later which stated that sodium had no effect on blood pressure. 10 years later the researchers published a follow up which now stated that sodium intake had no relationship to either coronary heart disease or death. This was a thorn in the side of those who had been promoting the low salt adage. It was quickly brushed aside.

A study called 'Intersalt' was designed by some of the foremost proponents of a low salt diet to be the study that resolved any of the remaining questions over the salt, blood pressure and it's heart disease link. It spanned ages 20 to 60 years old, involved 10,000 people from 52 different population groups and required the work and dedication of over 150 researchers. This was a costly and powerful research base! Interestingly it was published in the same 1988 issue of the British Medical Journal as the Scottish Heart study and it quickly became obvious that it had failed to confirm its primary hypothesis, the consistent link between salt and blood pressure. 48 of the 52 population groups showed no correlation between salt intake and blood pressure. Perhaps more embarrassingly for the researchers the group with the highest salt intake, Tianjin, China, at 14g per day had an almost identical healthy blood pressure to a Chicago African American population with only 6g salt per day, the lowest in the study. The only comparison they were able to make with blood pressure was total body mass and alcohol intake. 'Intersalts' leaders tried to find other weak associations to prove their original hypothesis and justify the costs of the study. However, two of the researchers involved with Intersalt, Kromhout and Hansson, said about their study:

'It did not show blood pressure increases if you eat a lot of salt.'

Nutrition's Playground

It is clear that the case for salt reduction is not without opposition. What is often considered a rock solid nutritional argument has been placed on shaky ground by some of the biggest studies ever done on salt and its effects on blood pressure and heart disease. Due to the volume of other studies that have suggested a link, the advice to lower salt intake still continues to be the overriding guidance provided.

We still need to answer the question asked earlier. Is the salt being traded today, the same as the salt that Jesus placed such a high value on? It should be noted that 99% of the world's research on salt is carried out on commercial table salt according to expert biochemist Dr Jacques De Langre. So what exactly is commercial salt? The truth is that commercial salt has gone through a series of significant changes that has altered it from what Nature intended. Most people generally think of salt as pure sodium chloride. Perhaps this is because the only thing that was available to them in the past was sodium chloride, available as table salt.

Sodium sanctification

A large majority of salt is produced by a method called vacuum pan salt refining. This basically involves the evaporation of brine. Before evaporation occurs it is common practice for the brine to be treated to remove minerals that can cause scaling within the evaporators and therefore affects its 'purity'. This chemical treatment of the brine causes a reduction in the levels of dissolved calcium, magnesium and sulphate. Sulphuric acid or chlorination may then be used to remove hydrogen sulphide whilst hydrochloric acid is then added to neutralise the remaining mixture. This 'purification' process is used as a way of creating high purity salt! There is truth in this fact. Manufacturers who use this method end up producing salt that is comprised of virtually 100% 'pure' sodium chloride, a form of salt. The remaining brine and chemical mixture is then subjected to forced circulation evaporation. This dries the brine allowing the salt to crystallise and precipitate but this is unable to remove all the fluid. The semi-crystallised salt is produced as slurry which then needs to be dried even further by centrifuging or vacuum drying. Then extreme heat is applied as it passes through the kiln where the water content is reduced to less than 0.05%.

Earlier in this chapter we looked at wheat and the extreme milling process that happens to create flour. An overview of the pasteurisation process illustrated the damaging effect this has upon the nutritional value of milk. The extracting and refining of sugar into an energy compound devoid of nutrients has had its toll on the human population. The processing of salt with the use of harsh acids, several applications of heat, centrifuge and finally drying, literally strips this natural compound of its life-giving properties. To produce a salty compound that is virtually 100% pure sodium chloride and is barely even a worthy imitation of what is naturally created in the oceans of the world as salt.

As previously noted, Weston A Price travelled the globe studying eating habits of indigenous populations that were separated from the Western world. With each of the 15 cultures he studied he sought out those who had come into contact with Western foods of commerce, typically white flour, pasteurised milk, refined sugar and processed salt. In every case, without exception, when these foods were introduced into healthy population groups deterioration in health soon followed. Large-scale manufacturing and processing has turned nature's valuable foodstuffs into life-draining,   immune-destroying,   nutrient-depleting

Nutrition's Playground

compounds! To remove these from the diet and seek out more nutritious options has got to be one of the first steps to regaining vitality and strength. However, to just remove the things that are unhealthy does not mean that we will develop optimal health. We must seek out and eat foods that provide vital nutrients in order to achieve this.

Nutrition's Playground

Step 4: Rustic Rejuvenation

The Latin root of the word 'rejuvenate' literally means young. Therefore, the definition of 'rejuvenates' is to make young again, to give new vigour or to restore to an original state. The Western population is in dire need of some rejuvenation, to restore our health to the state it once was. Apart from the blight of infectious disease through the centuries Western populations were considerably healthier several generations ago than they are now. Today life spans are greater than ever before, infectious diseases are in better control, but slowly developing chronic diseases, which were virtually unheard of only a century ago, now dominate the headlines and plague our society. In the words of Dr Arden Anderson, a world leading agronomist and medical doctor:

'There are many people in our modern society who are dead at 70, but are not buried until they are 90!'

This is not a 'once upon a time' story; only a few generations ago our society had a higher nutritional status and a better state of health than we witness today. Research clearly shows that even when health has been lost amongst a population group it can be gradually restored.

Dr. Francis M Pottenger ran a sanatorium in California and achieved great success in treating patients from respiratory

Nutrition's Playground

diseases like tuberculosis, asthma, emphysema and allergies. Whilst treating humans he also ran a 10-year experiment on a controlled population of cats. He divided them into 5 different groups and fed them different diets to observe the effects that each diet had on their health. The different diets involved raw meat and differing degrees of processed milk from pasteurised to sweetened condensed milk. Pottenger found that the only group that continued healthy from generation to generation were the group eating raw milk and meat. He observed that they had excellent bone structure, freedom from parasites, easy pregnancies and gentle dispositions. In the cats with the 2/3 processed food diets he reported a narrowing of the faces, crowded jaws, frail bones and weakened ligaments surrounding their joints. They were constantly plagued by parasites, developed diseases all across the spectrum of possibilities and suffered immensely in pregnancy. The female cats became very aggressive, whilst the males lost their vigour and became very docile. With each successive generation these problems became more pronounced until the experiment reached the fourth generation when young cats died before reaching adulthood and reproduction ceased altogether. Some critics of Pottenger's research claim that his work has no relevance to human beings because cats are carnivores whilst we are omnivores and would not thrive on raw meat and milk. In the many years that Pottenger ran his sanatorium he treated hundreds of human patients and observed in that time the same problems in his human patients as he did in his cats, often from the same cause, which is processed, nutrient deficient food. Although he had not intended for his cat studies to reflect on humans he did say:

'While no attempt will be made to correlate the changes in the animals studied with malformations found in humans, the similarity is so obvious that parallel pictures will suggest themselves.'

Nutrition's Playground

A profound side note for those who criticise Pottenger's work came from the research of Dr Price. The African Masai tribes, despite having omnivorous capabilities like all humans, lived off virtually nothing else but meat, raw milk and blood. These people were recorded as having outstanding bone structure, strength and immunity to disease! It may not be the ideal approach for everyone, but it certainly worked for the Masai. Dr Pottenger didn't end his studies once he had observed the slow degeneration and decline of his cats, but chose to see if he was able to gradually return them back to full health. He was able to accomplish this, but it took nearly twice as many generations to rear offspring with the same degree of health as the original cats. But the important point is that he was able to return the wretched feline offspring back to a high level of health. Dr Price also used the knowledge he had gained by studying primitive populations to help return human beings back to a higher state of health.

In Price's epic work, Nutrition and Physical Degeneration, he refers to a particular mother and her two daughters. The eldest girl was 10 years of age; she had an underdeveloped face and narrowed dental arches. She had pinched nostrils and as a result breathed mostly from her mouth even at rest when oxygen requirements are relatively low. He noted her disposition was very nervous and she often had a stooped posture. As it turns out her mother was fairly unhealthy during her pregnancy and had a troubled labour with her first daughter. Labour lasted 53 hours following which the mother was a partial invalid for several months after the birth. In the four years between the birth of the first child and the second Dr Price fed the mother on foods, which he knew from his primitive studies contained valuable fat-soluble nutrients and were rich in minerals. The foods included milk, green vegetables, seafood, organ meats, high vitamin cod liver oil and high vitamin butter oil. The birth of her second daughter was comparatively easy with a labour of only 3 hours and it had only a very slight impact on her strength and health and she was quickly able to focus on being a mother. The second child at the time of this being reported in the book was 6 years old, had broader and more complete facial structure and dental arches, breathed easily through her nose and had none of the nervous trouble of her older sister. It appears that as the health of the mother was restored with nutrient dense foods she more easily coped with the physical demands of childbirth and was able to produce a healthier child. This was only one of many case studies in Price's work highlighting the powerful effects of nutrient dense, primitive foods in rejuvenating health in previously deficient people. Nature knows what it takes to nurture health from the ground up! We just need to know how to tap into nature's life giving supply.

In the last chapter we noted the four dominant foods that Dr Weston A Price had discovered that had decimated modern health, namely white flour, pasteurised milk, refined white sugar and processed table salt. These all originally started out as foods that were distinctly locked in as part of nature's life giving food supply. How can we use these foods to contribute rather than rob us of our health?

Realising the Grains Potential

Archaeological evidence has shown that large-scale grain agriculture has been part of human existence for the best part of 18,000 years. During this significant time these plants have contributed to the sustaining of human life. Wheat, rye, barley, oats, and rice have all been the mainstay of one or more cultures in recorded history. Despite these grains being a part of the human food chain for so long it has only been

Nutrition's Playground

since the late 1800's that significant evidence of chronic degeneration has become apparent. The role that grains play in contributing to chronic degeneration has much more to do with the changes in the methods of production and large scale processing than it has with the actual grains. In the previous chapter large-scale grain manufacture was discussed in detail and many of the problems associated with steel roller mills, refining and the Chorleywood bread making process were exposed. The obvious question that comes to mind is how were grains traditionally prepared to maximise their nutritional content and support life?

Using the whole of the grain is a vital step in maximising the nutrient content of the grain. Remember that commercially processed 'whole grain' flour has actually been refined and separated into its component parts and then controlled amounts of bran and germ added back into the white refined flour. Despite this the high temperatures generated during roller milling have oxidised many of the vitamins and phytochemicals within the grain, robbing much of the valuable nutrient content.

Phytochemicals are beneficial chemical compounds that are naturally produced by plants which individually and synergistically support antioxidant, anti-inflammatory, anticancer and health preservation pathways in the body. Scientists have identified literally thousands of phytochemicals. Although our understanding of these compounds is in its infancy much of the research that has been done has already proven the vital role they play in our health. The bran and germ comprise only 15-17% of a grain of wheat, but over 80% of the phytochemicals, nutrients and many minerals are contained within these components. The inclusion of freshly ground whole flour in preference to refined will greatly increase the potential nutritive value.

Nutrition's Playground

However, it should also be recognised that many of these important compounds are not freely extracted by the digestive tract even though they are present. This is because many phytochemicals and minerals are 'bound' within the bran and germ as a protective mechanism to store the nutrients within the grain in readiness for the time of germination. In the previous chapter these binding compounds were identified as phytic acid, tannins, enzyme inhibitors, complex sugars, gluten and other hardy proteins. Simply milling whole grains unfortunately does not unlock these nutrients, as they will remain bound to the fibrous parts of the grain, which simply pass through the digestive tract without absorption into the blood stream.

If these health-promoting nutrients are bound within the bran and germ in readiness for germination then it becomes apparent when germination occurs the nutrients are released from their 'bound' form to aid growth of the plant. Therefore, one way of ensuring that the nutrients are available for digestion is to consume sprouted grain products or breads, where germination has occurred prior to milling the grains. The drawback of this method is the time taken to sprout the grains prior to their use. There are commercially produced sprouted breads that can be purchased, but understand that many of the nutrients that are made available through germination are prone to oxidative damage. The more time that has passed since the grains have been milled, both before and after the bread has been made, the greater the chances of a reduced nutrient content.

Drawing the nutrients out

Traditionally a more effective method was used that did not sprout the grains prior to milling, but was able to free the 'bound' nutrients whilst significantly increasing the digestibility of the grains. This method involved a fermentation process that helped to make foodstuffs more digestible and nutrient dense. Different cultures have slightly different fermentation methods and they don't always involve the use of grains. In Europe grains were traditionally sour leavened to produce sourdough breads. Sour leavening is the process of mixing flour; rye seems to work best, with warm water and introducing a lactic acid bacteria culture to the medium to allow fermentation to take place over several days. This type of fermentation does not produce alcohol; rather these bacteria produce lactic acid, which has a slightly sour taste, hence, the name. In recent years, perhaps due to the alarming increase in gluten intolerance, there has been a sizeable amount of scientific research focused on the souring or fermentation of grains and its effects on the body.

In 2006 a study published in Letters in Applied Microbiology found that several strains or types of bacteria played an important part in sourdough fermentation. They observed that the lactic acid bacteria and another strain called pediococci both fed off the protein in gluten to obtain nitrogen for growth. This serves two very valuable purposes in bread preparation. Firstly in metabolising this necessary nitrogen source the bacteria release carbon dioxide, which serves to leaven or raise the bread without the need of baker's yeast. Secondly as the study observed the:

'bacteria strains isolated from sourdough are proteolytically active on gluten.'

This basically means that gluten is gradually used up and removed from the grain mixture during sourdough fermentation. This is incredibly beneficial for individuals who suffer from gluten intolerance. Another study published in 2007 in Applied and Environmental Microbiology also investigated the effects of sourdough lactic acid bacteria on gluten, but particularly focused on the tolerance of sourdough bread on those suffering from Celiac disease. Celiac is an autoimmune response to the presence of gliadin, a protein found in gluten of the triticum family of grains. The Triticeae family includes typical wheat, spelt, durum, barley and rye. The bowel becomes inflamed when gliadin is present making nutrient absorption very difficult, creating discomfort and often diarrhoea. In Europe it is estimated that the prevalence of Celiac disease is around 2% of the population. The 2007 research study stated that sourdough fermentation using lactic acid bacteria:

'may be considered an efficient approach to eliminate gluten toxicity.'

The scientists found that the bacteria absorbed the gliadin proteins and metabolised them, lowering the total reactive gluten to minimal levels. In cases where they fermented the grains for 48 hours they found the reactive gluten levels dropped to levels of less than 20 parts per million. This is the level stated by the World Health Organisation and the Food and Agricultural Organisation as meeting the requirements for 'gluten free'!

The typical advice offered to those with gluten intolerance or Celiac disease is to eat a gluten free diet for the rest of their life. Not only is this very challenging with today's supermarket culture, but this usually leads people to eat highly processed foods made out of gluten free grains or flour like oats, millet, rice flour, potato flour, soya flour or gram flour. This may reduce or completely stop the occurrence of gluten reactions but may not lead to a nutrient dense diet that will support health. Tradition seems to have an alternative answer in the production of sourdough breads and other fermented foods. Souring or bacterial fermentation naturally removes the gluten whilst breaking down mineral blocking phytic acid so that the rich mineral compounds are freed for absorption into the body. In a way the lactic acid bacteria predigest the grains for us making them much easier to digest and absorb ourselves, without the unwanted irritation to the gut wall.

Sourdough breads may not always be the answer for those suffering from gluten intolerance or Celiac disease, but it is certainly beneficial for many who have tried it. Mike had suffered from irritable bowel for some years and had been advised by his doctor to avoid all wheat and gluten containing grains. He had followed this advice and found that he rarely suffered the bloating, nausea, fatigue and chronic diarrhoea he had become accustomed to in the past. He did his best to avoid gluten where possible, but occasionally learned the hard way when the symptoms came raging back. Often upon closer inspection he would find gluten-containing ingredients in the food product and have to cross another item off his future shopping list. His wife learned about the benefits of sourdough bread and decided to give it a try. She followed the instructions carefully, cultured her own sourdough starter over several days of fermentation, prepared the bread and allowed a long proving or rising time before baking the loaf. Mike tried the bread and loved the taste. He waited for the familiar symptoms to kick in. 1 hour, 2 hours, 3, 6, and even 24 hours later there was a total absence of the distinct reactions he had tolerated during the previous years. This proved to be a fantastic breakthrough as Mike had sorely missed bread and that fresh baked taste.

Several months have passed since that first experience and Mike has rarely had any negative response from sourdough bread. Why rarely? The only time he has reacted is when his wife was short on time or was too eager to cook the bread and did not allow the bread to prove for long enough. If the proving time was only 2-3 hours it seems the lactic acid bacteria had not yet fed and removed all the gluten and as a result Mike experienced the uncomfortable symptoms. However, when the proving time was at least 6 hours or longer he always enjoyed the bread with no negative reaction.

A suitable proving time period is essential for minimising gluten and ensuring the grain or flour contained within the bread has been properly 'pre-digested' by the lactic acid bacteria. It appears that a time period of between 8-12 hours is suitably long enough to prove the bread and allow it to rise whilst still giving the bacteria sufficient time to feed on the gluten. This will vary somewhat based on the ambient temperature and the activity of the bacteria. Proving time is typically longer in the winter and shorter in the summer months of the year.

Real Milk

Pasteurisation has only been robbing milk of its life force since its widespread introduction in the early 1900s in the USA. Pasteurisation began en masse in the UK and other parts of Europe around the 1940s. Archaeological evidence indicates that peoples north of the Red Sea used antelope milk as a food source as early as 30,000 years ago. There were many other cultures breeding and using animals for milk literally thousands of years before the planting and use of grains in mass agriculture. This means that for 29,900 of those years the milk that was being used and ingested by humans in various populations all over the globe was raw, untreated, full fat, natural milk! Yet today the reaction by many when I tell them that I drink raw milk, as does my wife and children is usually one of confusion and concern. Why and how have we become afraid of nature's first and unique foodstuff, raw milk? Surely almost 30,000 years of time across millions of people is a broad enough 'experiment' to consider a food safe and of substantial value to our health? In order to satisfy even the most determined Doubting Thomas it would be prudent to investigate the beneficial effects of raw milk and under what circumstances it is safe to drink this essential food.

A mothering cow produces raw milk as stand alone sustenance for her newborn calf. It makes complete sense that this self produced fluid needs to contain a wide variety of nutrients in sufficient amounts to not only maintain the life of the young, but to promote growth and full health. Raw milk contains all major nutrient components such as fats, proteins, carbohydrates, vitamins, minerals, water and enzymes. It serves as complete nutrition for the calf. This admittedly is not complete nutrition for a human being, but the many nutritive components are in dense concentration, therefore making it highly beneficial for humans as well. The following section provides a comparison between raw and pasteurised milk:

Comparison between Raw and Pasteurised milk

Enzymes:
Raw - All fully available
Pasteurised - Anywhere from 0 -10% remaining.

Protein:
Raw - 100% available, all 22 amino acids, including the 9 that are essential
Pasteurised - lysine and tyrosine are altered by heat with serious loss of metabolic availability. This results in making the whole protein complex less available for tissue repair and rebuilding.

Nutrition's Playground

Fats:
Raw - All 18 saturated and unsaturated fatty acids metabolically available. If grass fed - contains valuable conjugated linoleic acid (CLA)
Pasteurised - Altered by heat, especially the 10 essential unsaturated fats.

Vitamins:
Raw - All 100% available.
Pasteurised - Loss of vitamins A, D, E and K can run as high as 66%. Losses on water-soluble vitamins are affected by heat and can run from 38% to 80%. Vitamin C loss usually exceeds 50%

Carbohydrates:
Raw - Easily utilized in metabolism
Pasteurised - Tests indicate that heat has made some changes making elements less available metabolically.

Minerals:
Raw - All 100% metabolically available. Major mineral components are calcium, chlorine, magnesium, phosphorus, potassium, sodium and sulphur. Vital trace minerals, all 24 or more, 100% available.
Pasteurised - Calcium is altered by heat and losses may run 50% or more, depending on pasteurisation temperature. Losses in other essential minerals, because one mineral usually acts synergistically with another element. There is a loss of enzymes that serve as leaders in assimilating minerals.

NOTE: Bacteria growth in Raw Milk increases very slowly, because of the friendly acid-forming bacteria (nature's antiseptic) retards the growth of invading organisms (bacteria). Usually keeps for several weeks when under refrigeration and will sour instead of rot. Bacteria growth will

Nutrition's Playground

be geometrically rapid after pasteurisation and homogenisation. Gradually turns rancid in a few days, and then decomposes.

Adapted from information produced at www.realmilk.com

Revelations from science

The following section is not intended to be a comprehensive review of all the information supporting raw milk, but a selection of some of the positive lesser-known research. There are many studies that have shown the superiority of raw milk over pasteurised milk from a health perspective.

In 1917 The American Journal of Diseases of Children reported that raw milk had been proven to protect against flu, diphtheria and pneumonia as well as having a preventative effect with regards to scurvy. Young children who had developed scurvy after several months of drinking pasteurised milk were soon cured after changing to raw milk.

A study published in the magazine, Nature, in 1931 involved 20,000 school children in Scotland. 5000 kids were fed ¾ pint of raw milk daily, 5000 were fed the same amount of pasteurised milk and the remaining children were not fed milk and were to serve as a control to compare the other two groups against. The report that was published in March of 1931 stated that there was no difference in the growth or weight in either group. However, the very next month in the April copy of Nature, two scientists published a critical evaluation of the study and caught out the bias in the original conclusion. They identified that the results actually showed a significant increase in growth in the boys who were drinking raw milk in comparison to those drinking pasteurised.

Nutrition's Playground

In January of 1933 it was published in the Ohio Agricultural Experiment Station Bulletin that much more favourable calcium balances were achieved with the intake of several months of raw milk feeding compared to pasteurised milk feeding. This was also confirmed by the Lancet in 1937, when studying chilblains, it was found that the higher calcium values obtained through using raw milk, compared to pasteurised, virtually eliminated the incidence of this disease in children.

In 1937 the British medical journal, The Lancet, published a study that concluded children fed raw milk had a higher resistance to tuberculosis (TB) than those fed pasteurised milk. The same study also indicated that raw milk prevented tooth decay.

In July 1938 The Drug and Cosmetic Industry published a report that identified that pathological organisms do not proliferate and grow in raw milk, but grow rapidly in pasteurised milk.

In 1944 The Annual review of Biochemistry reported that the cream from raw milk was beneficial in preventing stiffness in joints.

In more recent years in 1999 the Lancet published a study that demonstrated that raw milk protects against asthma and allergic skin problems.

An excellent study published in 2006 in the Journal of Allergy and Clinical Immunology reported that childhood consumption of high quality raw milk resulted in large reductions in the incidence of asthma, eczema and hay fever. Blood tests revealed that drinking raw milk reduced the levels of histamine, an internal chemical stimulant for allergic reaction, by as much as 50%.

Since pasteurisation became the normal method of mass milk production scientific research on the benefits of raw milk virtually stopped. This happened in the late 1940's and from that point there was a period of many years where little or no research was carried out on raw milk except to highlight the need to pasteurise because of harmful toxins present in raw milk. As you can see above some research has begun again and surprisingly to some it has revealed positive evidence.

Raw milk, but different

One problem that is rarely pointed out by the big dairies or those who pronounce the terrible ills of raw milk is that there are two types of raw milk! The first is raw milk produced by cows in perfect health and living as Mother Nature intended on a diet of freshly growing, green grass. I will refer to this as fresh, unprocessed milk from this point on. The second type is raw milk from cattle that are mass-produced and bred for maximum milk production in large, commercial ventures on a diet of grains and processed feed. This milk will be referred to as commercial raw milk from this point onwards.

The American Food and Drug Administration have said that drinking raw milk is like playing Russian roulette with your health. This would most certainly be true of commercial raw milk. The cattle are in a much less healthy condition as a result of the stress and the burden of meeting overwhelming milk demands from greedy farmers and dairy companies. The excess grains, corn, soy, citrus peel cake and bakery waste routinely offered as feed cause a shift of pH in the stomachs of the cattle, creating an acid environment which encourages the proliferation of harmful bacteria. This the reason why

Nutrition's Playground

commercial farmers need to add antibiotics into cattle feed on a regular basis to keep the pathogenic bacteria at bay. The cattle are bred to produce three times the milk of the old fashioned dairy cow. This volume of production draws heavily on the reserves of the mother cow, diluting the vitamin and mineral content of the milk considerably. The lack of beneficial bacteria in the milk allows for the increase in harmful bacteria instead. So drinking watery, low vitamin and mineral content milk combined with an increase in unchecked, pathogenic bacteria would certainly qualify for comparison to Russian roulette. This is NOT the milk that one should drink, hence the only option with this kind of milk, to increase safety for consumption, is to pasteurise the product. It is more productive and profitable to produce milk in this way and then to teach the general public that pasteurisation is a must for all milk.

Fresh, unprocessed milk comes from happy, contented cows that live on a diet of green grass. This is as it should be. Then the cattle are healthy inside as well as out and do not require a constant dosing with antibiotics. Their gut flora is beneficial to the health of the cow and serves to enrich the milk, which becomes a natural probiotic, which in turn enriches the gut flora of the drinker, be it calf or human. The cow produces an appropriate amount of milk rich in beneficial fats (like anti carcinogenic CLA), building proteins, vitamins (A, D, E & K), minerals, enzymes and good bacteria. This is a life sustaining drink that can support health for generations, providing the standards of production are maintained.

Probably one of the biggest proponents of fresh, unprocessed milk was a man by the name of Charles Sanford Porter, MD. Dr. Porter published a book called Milk Diet as a Remedy for Chronic Disease in 1905 which progressed through a further 11 editions until the last one was published in 1923. Porter marvelled at having helped over 18,000 patients who had received treatment from him during 37 years of practise with his milk cure. Porter, a believer in food as key to disease correction, said:

'A good food is a good remedy, and, as disease is only a disturbance of the mechanism of nutrition, it is only natural that the use of milk in ill health should be almost as old as its use as a food in health.'

Porter emphasized that milk as a root cause of good health MUST come from clean, healthy cattle and that no degree of processing was acceptable as it was then likely to cause ill health in preference to good health. Porter recalled receiving a letter in 1913 from a man named Mr Kitzele who had suffered an injury in his youth that meant he could not eat any solid food and had been living exclusively on fresh, unprocessed milk ever since. Porter sought him out and in 1921 received further information on this individual. He had been living on milk alone for almost 50 years and in that time had never spent a single day in bed sick and was as healthy and strong as any man doing office work! This story is not relayed as a suggestion to live exclusively on fresh, unprocessed milk in order to be healthy, but to illustrate that in this extreme circumstance exclusive milk intake had the nutrient density to keep this man healthy for over 50 years.

Milk for health

The industry has relied for many years on the knowledge that dairy foods are a rich source of calcium. A 14 year study of nearly 1000 men and women published in the British medical journal, The Lancet, in 1988 stated

'The only factor consistently and significantly associated with the risk of hip fracture was dietary calcium: the risk of hip fracture

Nutrition's Playground

decreased in relation to increasing levels of calcium intake in both men and women.'

This study was run looking at pasteurised milk consumption and as we have stated earlier calcium losses can run as high as 50% during processing. One can only wonder how much stronger the association between bone density and dietary calcium intake would have been if fresh, unprocessed milk had been used. Despite this there are numerous studies indicating dairy produce as a good source of much needed calcium.

In 1996 a Finnish study was published in the British Journal of Cancer concluding 25 years of research involving over 4500 women. They had divided the women into 5 groups governed by their occupations, agriculture, industry, services, white collar and housewives. They found that milk intake was inversely associated with a lower incidence of breast cancer! The agricultural group had by a large margin the lowest incidence of breast cancer throughout the study. These were all ladies who lived on farms, so it is reasonable to assume, though not documented, that they were drinking fresh, unprocessed milk as is the norm and tradition on most natural farms throughout the region. The lower breast cancer rate may have been due to the higher levels of the nutrient CLA, which has been shown in several studies to have powerful anti-cancer properties.

Another important reason for the regular consumption of fresh, unprocessed milk is to receive the benefits of the healthy bacteria that naturally flourish in high quality milk. It is now understood that almost 70% of our immune response comes from our gut. This is mainly down to the natural balance that should exist between the good, bad and neutral bacteria. The ideal scenario being that the good lactic acid producing bacteria maintain a sufficient population to lower the pH of the gut enough to prevent the bad bacteria from flourishing. An appropriate balance will also contribute towards digesting carbohydrates, positively influencing cholesterol, synthesizing certain vitamins and breaking down enzymes, proteins and fibre.

This is the basis for the emerging and powerful market in probiotic drinks. These products were introduced to the UK market in the mid 1990s and flourished as well as the bacteria they are deemed to promote in the gut! By 2006 the probiotic drinks market was worth over £227 million in the UK with over 830 million bottles being sold annually. So are these drinks actually good for us? Despite the presence of large amounts of added sugar and flavourings there is some evidence to suggest that some of the larger brands patented bacteria can help prevent diarrhoea in children and temporarily aid immunity. However, the levels of bacteria per bottle are fairly low and tests show that about half will die or be lost on the journey through the digestive system. Perhaps a more important question is where has this vast need for boosting your gut bacterial flora come from? It may be due to either a lack of good gut bacteria, or an unhealthy increase in the pathogenic bacteria in our guts. The ever increasing amounts of sugar and sugar alternatives in our modern diet will certainly contribute to the latter as these highly refined carbohydrates serve as excellent fuel to the pathogenic and yeast fermenting bacteria creating undesirable conditions in the gut.

Prior to the mid 1990s and the grand introduction of the probiotic drink there must have been foods that contributed and aided the natural balance of the gut flora. This type of imbalance has only been identified as a problem in more recent years. The inclusion of certain unprocessed fruits and vegetables and some grains can contribute to the natural

Nutrition's Playground

bacteria balance in the gut. Despite many years promoting these 'healthy' foods, many in the population still fail to ingest sufficient amounts. Fresh, unprocessed milk or yoghurt is perhaps amongst the best and longest standing natural probiotics there are. But since big dairy began blanket pasteurisation this has forcibly removed the premier probiotic from our readily available foods. Pasteurisation not only destroys any pathogenic bacteria in milk but also destroys all the beneficial bacteria, completely eradicating its role as a probiotic!

The regular consumption of organic, completely grass fed, antibiotic free, unprocessed cow's milk and natural yoghurt should play a vital role in the health of many in the population. At present it is strengthening only a small percentage because it is not as readily available as it should be.

It is a basic right to be able to choose the foods you would like to eat and readily have access to them. Adults currently have the freedom to choose whether they smoke or not, though it may not be as socially acceptable as it once was. There are volumes of evidence about the dangers of smoking and how it causes many diseases, yet provided you are old enough it is readily available. It is true commercial raw milk has been produced in conditions that are not always conducive of good health and for human safety there is an argument for controlling its production and maybe even pasteurisation. The historical fear of raw milk is linked to the ravages of a bacterial disease called tuberculosis (TB). Many people suffered from this terrible infection in the early part of the 20th century and thousands of deaths resulted. It seems one of the most convenient scapegoats at the time was to blame it on raw milk in the cities, rather than the dirty and cramped living conditions that many were subjected to. The disease was not fully understood then, but now it seems highly unlikely that TB was passed on to humans through milk. TB affects the area of the body that it comes into contact with, and most human TB was contracted in the lungs, causing respiratory problems. Today it is easily treated, but at the turn of the century it was difficult to control. If TB had been contracted from raw milk it would have been the bovine strain of TB not the human strain and the bacteria would have affected the intestinal tract not the lungs. A deeper investigation of TB is needed to fully understand the workings of the disease and why it is highly unlikely that raw milk ever really caused TB and is unlikely to ever cause TB in humans where good safety practises are present. A full understanding of TB is beyond the scope and purpose of this book.

Creamy, fresh, unprocessed milk is a nutrient dense, health promoting elixir, restorative to the body and as natural as Mother Nature intended it to be. This most desirable form of milk is available in our Western society, but often there are unjustifiable restrictions or limitations to its sale. There should not be fear, but a love of this delicious super food. The nutritive benefits of raw milk far outweigh any risks providing high quality, organic, grass fed, healthy cows, particularly traditional Jersey and Guernsey breeds, are sought for as the source of this outstanding food.

Indulge your Sweet Tooth

It is well documented that refined sugars have many damaging side effects on human metabolism. They have been found to

- increase dental decay

Nutrition's Playground

- upset blood sugar levels

- stimulate reactive hypoglycaemia

- contribute to insulin resistance

- affect behavioural problems

- fuel hyperactivity in children

- increase anxiety

- suppress the immune system

- trigger binge eating

- boost Candida growth

- aggravate symptoms of PMS

- promote fat storage

Despite all of these concerning effects we must also recognise that the human body does have a mechanism for sweet taste and may even at times crave foods that will provide for this. In the last chapter it was highlighted that refined sugar intake has rocketed in recent years with people ingesting huge amounts on a regular basis. This has likely conditioned the population to much higher levels of sweetness than would naturally be sought after by the body.

Research by Princeton University suggests that it is even possible to develop an addiction to sugar where cravings become so intense it becomes impossible to give it up as

Nutrition's Playground

dependence upon the substance sets in. It is important to understand that negative behaviours are linked to highly processed or refined sugars. Nature has provided us with naturally sweet substances which when taken in moderate amounts can help satisfy a healthy desire for sweetness whilst still providing suitable nutrition for the body.

Bee-autifully sweet

Evidence of the use of honey in society dates back many thousands of years. Ancient Egyptian writings referring to honey date back as far as 5500 BC. There are many cultures around the globe from regions of India to the Australian Aborigines who prized honey for its taste and nutritive qualities. Hunter-gatherers were known to be able to collect honey freely from the hive by smoking out the bees beforehand. Getting stung in the process, though this was rare, was seen as a worthwhile sacrifice to enjoy the beautiful honey contained within. Yet this delicacy did not cause an abundance of dental cavities amongst the people who sought it on occasion. Perhaps that is the reason why, it was only enjoyed from time to time. Today honey is available freely in the supermarkets from many different sources and many different types. It can come from all around the globe from New Zealand to Argentina. There are several types, clear 'runny' honey, thick opaque honey, solid 'set' honey, organic honey and manuka honey are just a few that are usually found on the shop shelves. Despite this great range of products, do we get in these jars what nature intended to sustain the life of the bee?

Honey is the nectar drawn from flowers transported by bees back to the hive where it is deposited into hexagonal wax cells to provide nourishment to the hive, particularly the young. The nectar begins to change through enzymatic action

Nutrition's Playground

and the warmth in the hive, which gradually evaporates excess fluid converting the nectar into honey. The enzymes that assist in the breakdown of nectar originate from the saliva of the bees, resulting in the splitting of sucrose, a double sugar, into its two component parts, fructose and glucose. These single sugars require almost no digestion and are able to be absorbed into the blood without much effort from the digestive system. Honey varies a lot with the region, seasons and the flowers in the area that the bees draw nectar from. On average honey consists of about 35-40% fructose and 30-35% glucose. The remainder is made up of about 20% water, traces of pollen, propolis, some wax, proteins, enzymes, gums, vitamins and minerals. Propolis is a substance produced from collected plant resins that is used like bee glue to construct and repair cracks in the hive. The amount of gum present usually has a direct influence on the thickness of the final honey.

In many cases commercial honey purchased at the supermarket has been through a refining process. It is common for it to have been heated during extraction, which destroys many of the enzymes and oxidises the vitamins. It is often filtered several times for 'purity', which usually removes the pollen, propolis, waxes and any dust or mould. This leaves behind mostly the sugary component without the nutritive compounds that should co-exist with this food. The processing of honey strips it back to a food that is likely to upset our body's blood sugar levels but more importantly has lost many of its beneficial properties.

Honey should be processed as little as possible, if at all. In Russia beekeepers have been noted for their health and longevity, although many factors are likely to be at work here, traditionally this is said to be due to their custom of eating the honey remains from the bottom of the hive. This 'bottom' honey contained high levels of what would today be seen as impurities; pollen, propolis, wax and even bee parts. To obtain the health benefits of honey it should not be heated at all and filtered as little as possible. There have been many health claims made regarding raw, unfiltered honey.

Science so sweet

Some of these have been scientifically tested whilst others are more to do with tradition and folklore.

A study published in Chemical-Biological Interactions in 1992 found that certain compounds contained within propolis had strong anti-cancer properties when tested on colon cancer cells.

A 1990 study by Gribel and Pashinskii demonstrated that honey had moderate anti-tumour effects on five different strains of rat and mouse tumours.

Researchers from Waikato University in New Zealand found that honey was able to completely stop the growth of certain bacteria that are known to cause gastric ulcers. Another physician called Dr Schacht, of Wiesbaden, claims to have cured many hopeless cases of gastric and intestinal ulcers using raw honey and no surgical intervention.

Bacteriologists further tested the effects of honey against germs that cause typhoid, bronco-pneumonia and dysentery and found that the cultures were completely killed off in the presence of raw honey.

When eaten with other sources of carbohydrates, like toast or porridge, the enzymes in honey have been shown to aid in

Nutrition's Playground

the natural breakdown and digestion of these more complex carbohydrates.

Research involving 17,862 patients that focused on using raw honey to treat respiratory problems found that the majority had their symptoms disappear or significantly improve. 64% of those with chronic bronchitis, 62% of those with asthmatic bronchitis and 56% of those with sinusitis had a complete absence of symptoms following treatment.

Dr William G Peterson from Oklahoma, USA, has cared for literally thousands of patients with allergies using raw honey as one of his treatments. He said 'It must be raw honey, because raw honey contains all the pollen, dust and moulds that cause 90% of all allergies. What happens is that the patient builds up immunity to pollen, dust or mould that is causing his trouble in the first place. I know the customer wants good, clear strained honey, and that's fine, but for health reasons raw, *unfiltered* [my emphasis] honey is what we need.' Other health claims include improvement of anaemia, rheumatic arthritis, hay fever, skin burns and overall digestive capacity.

Honey, as you can see, has a myriad of health enhancing benefits. Don't get caught up with the supermarket commercial varieties, seek out and find locally produced, raw, unfiltered honey where possible. Then you can receive the real health benefits rather than just a huge sugar rush. Even though raw honey is a truly nutritious food, perhaps we should remember that the hunter-gatherers only ate this prized food occasionally. Enjoy it, but do not over indulge.

Nutrition's Playground

Maple syrup is another very beneficial sweetener that has been replaced by refined sugar, much to our loss. In fact maple syrup production is now about 20% of what is was at the beginning of the 20th century. When the heavy taxes placed on the importation of refined sugar began to be significantly reduced it made it easier for the masses to purchase and it could be produced on a very large scale. The majority of the world's maple syrup is produced in North America, particularly in Quebec, which generates about 75% of total global production. Traditionally maple syrup was made by boring a hole through the bark of the sugar maple tree and placing a tap into the wood and then collecting the sap in a bucket over a period of time. The sap is very watery and only contains about 2-3% sugar, making it virtually tasteless. Once a sufficient amount of sap was collected it was necessary to boil off large amounts of the water to concentrate the sugars and help produce the beautiful, distinct flavour it is renowned for.

Modern sap production

Today in almost all cases buckets have been replaced by continuous plastic piping that leads to the 'sugar shack' or to holding tanks at a lower altitude, hence using gravity for collection. Maple sap is best collected from February to April when the temperature in Canada and North America usually varies from freezing nights to warm days. This undulating temperature causes the tree to draw up water from the ground and creates stem pressure from within, ideal for sap collecting. Today rather than just boiling the syrup down, reverse osmosis has been introduced to remove 80% of the water. This helps to reduce energy consumption and decreases the exposure of the syrup to high temperatures. In a typical 6 week season a single maple tree is likely to yield about 40 litres of sap, which sounds like a considerable amount. However, once the sap is concentrated into the final product that 40 litres will only give rise to a single litre of pure maple syrup!

This means that manufacture is a slow process, which explains the higher prices for pure maple syrup over the imitation syrups. The imitation syrups contain virtually no maple syrup if any at all and are predominantly made of high fructose corn syrup, a heavily refined sugar that is detrimental to our health. A simple internet search on the dangers of high fructose corn syrup will unearth plenty of information on the subject. The imitation product fortunately cannot, by law, be labelled 'maple syrup' and therefore can be easily avoided.

Maple syrup at only 260kcal/100g contains fewer calories than refined sugar at 390kcal/100g and honey at 300kcal/100g. Maple syrup is also very rich in minerals, particularly the trace mineral manganese at over 150% of the government daily amount and zinc at 42% of the daily amount. Manganese is a powerful antioxidant whilst zinc plays vital roles in protecting the heart and supporting reproductive function. Seek out organic, pure maple syrup where possible to ensure no harmful chemicals have been concentrated into the syrup.

The Real Salt Diet

Salt is a naturally occurring compound that is found in the sea, the soil, the rocks and even small amounts within the food we eat. Although it is present naturally in food, Mother Nature is not conspiring to try and poison us by boosting our salt levels and increasing blood pressure and heart disease. In the previous chapter we discussed the salt hypothesis and highlighted some of the major studies that have been unable to draw any conclusion to pin salt down as a culprit in the

Nutrition's Playground

aetiology of disease. The Scottish Heart Health Study and Intersalt, two of the largest salt investigations in modern history received significant financial investment and were still unable to make any convincing link between salt and hypertension. In April 1997 The New England Journal of Medicine published a study called the Dietary Approaches to Stop Hypertension (DASH). The DASH study guidelines are often quoted to support the reduction of salt and fat whilst increasing fruit and vegetables as a successful method of lowering blood pressure. However, when the methodology and results of the study are actually investigated it becomes apparent that the study did not prove all of those factors. In fact it even suggests that salt may not be a player in reducing blood pressure at all. The study looked at several groups of people, including those with mild and severe hypertension and applied a DASH protocol to varying degrees, but the one thing they kept constant across all diets was the level of salt intake. The level that blood pressure decreased varied across the dietary groups, but as salt was constant in all groups it had nothing to do with the reduction in blood pressure. Yet the advice at the conclusion of the DASH investigation suggested further research needed to be done, but in the mean time salt reduction was wise! Where did that come from? Their study certainly didn't provide any evidence to back up this little gem. It sometimes seems that regardless of the findings of substantial science that salt has been tarred with a black brush that is difficult to clean up. What happened to being innocent until proven guilty? Or perhaps in this case being allowed retribution in the court of appeal! Fortunately there has been research done in defence of salt.

First it needs to be understood that a wide variety of factors have been found to influence blood pressure, therefore making it difficult to single out a culprit. Sodium plays a role in maintaining blood volume, whilst potassium influences the

98

Nutrition's Playground

walls of the blood vessels to dilate or constrict and calcium helps the smooth muscle within the blood vessel walls to contract when needed to help blood distribution. Each one of these minerals can influence blood pressure.

It is also well known that the amount of food that we eat has some bearing. If you increase the amount of calories within your diet the body's nervous system responds by constricting blood vessels slightly and therefore increasing the internal pressure. A reduction in the number of calories ingested has the opposite effect, where vessels dilate and pressure drops. It is highly likely that when individuals become conscious of their salt intake they are also on a weight management diet of some kind, which often means a reduction of calories. Does the calorie or salt reduction cause the pressure decrease that may be observed? All of these variables are complicated a little more when we realise that each factor differs from person to person across gender, age and even ethnic origin! It is not so simple. This is why there is still debate, even today, amongst the scientific community about whether or not salt causes high blood pressure and therefore could be bad for your heart.

Defending salt

In the previous chapter Dr Jacques De Langre received a brief introduction as an expert who had spent over 30 years studying salt and its benefits. He is one of the foremost voices in the world for promotion of salt as a vital health food rather than a devil waiting to pounce. Dr De Langre claims that 99% of all research on salt is performed on commercial table salt, which has been highly processed as described in the previous chapter. He agrees with the fact that refined salt has been shown to have some adverse side effects

Nutrition's Playground

'Yet, a salt free diet has problems of its own. They're in a scientific rut. Neither approach, taking refined salt, nor avoiding it is the answer.'

It is strange that medicine seems to take a blanket view of small indicators in scientific literature, believing that if the tiny effects identified in research studies are spread across the population at large this will lead to more substantial effects in the health of thousands of people. This follows some logical train of thought, but has not been backed up by its application in the instance of salt reduction across the masses. In a 1991 issue of the scientific journal Hypertension, Dr John Laragh expressed his concerns about the advice for the population at large to be restricting their salt intake. He said that reducing salt as a preventative treatment for hypertension:

'...must remain an interesting speculation, without enough evidence to justify its conclusion as part of a national programme.'

This low salt mantra has been pushed for 30 years and yet we still see significant numbers with elevated blood pressure, cardiovascular disease and stroke. The British Food Standards Agency has recently indicated that most food processing manufacturers have taken on board the advice to lower salt intake in their products and this has clearly changed in recent years. However disease rates have changed very little despite this reduction. Dr De Langre puts a different slant on it. Instead of always highlighting the problems of taking in too much salt he reminds us how vital salt is for our existence.

'You can't function without salt. You can't digest food without salt. Your heart can't function. Your adrenal glands can't function. Your kidneys can't function. Sodium is the dominant cat ion in the circulating blood plasma and tissue fluids. People forget that

Nutrition's Playground

everyone was born in a salty solution, our mother's amniotic fluid. This is probably the best biological proof we have that cellular structure is enhanced by salt. The amniotic fluid is a salty mini ocean for the foetus.'

It seems this everlasting mantra to avoid salt has been taken too far. If salt was so bad for us then why do hospitals feed the sick and infirm on intravenous drips that contain saline solutions? This is because salt is highly beneficial for healing and aids the repairing of human tissues. Seawater is a very complex chemical solution that contains 84 of the 103 known elements. These elements are vital to the maintaining of a suitable environment for sea life. In the 1900's a medical doctor ran a simple experiment to demonstrate the problems of using pure sodium chloride rather than full spectrum sea salt. He prepared a fish tank but used pure sodium chloride and ensured the concentration of this refined salt was the same as in seawater. All the fish died shortly after being put in the tank. They could not live in an environment of diluted pure sodium chloride and neither can we. We may not live in the sea, but several salt scientists have referred to our blood stream as being like a mini ocean that nourishes and supports the human body from within. In the ocean sodium is buffered by many other chemicals, in our blood sodium is buffered and so our diet too should be buffered or protected against the effects of pure sodium chloride.

Nature's way

Natural unprocessed sea salt contains all the natural elements in the ocean. Unprocessed sea salt, hand harvested in Brittany in northern France is believed to be the finest in the world. The seawater is slowly precipitated through long lakes that allow particles and sediment to settle to the bottom whilst the surface water is directed into a series of concentrating ponds for 1-2 miles. The water becomes a beautiful blue and the wind and sun alone are used to dry the water out leaving the moist crystallised salts behind. No artificial heat is used at any stage which ensures that the remaining salt is still biologically active. Although unprocessed sea salt is still predominantly sodium chloride, it is the few percent of many other minerals that make the difference. About 1% of natural, unprocessed sea salt is magnesium and this gives the salt its slightly grey, moist appearance and texture. Magnesium is a water-hugging molecule. Most sea salts sold in supermarkets are pure white and dry, this is almost a guarantee that the magnesium levels are low or nonexistent. One of the vital roles of magnesium in the body is to scrounge around helping to remove excess sodium from the blood stream and remove it through the kidneys.

'It's one of the great nutritional paradoxes that you have to give (natural unprocessed) salt, in order to lower the level of (refined) salt in the tissues' My emphasis added

This is greatly beneficial as it actually contributes to the effective functioning of the circulatory system and bringing blood pressure to optimal levels. When a blood pressure lowering medication is taken it will only do one thing, that is lower the pressure within the system by forcing a change in the controlling mechanisms. Sometimes this can create problems of its own. Natural, unprocessed sea salt has the ability to return to centre whatever function is unbalanced within the internal 'mini ocean' of the body. De Langre claims that over the years he has had over 2000 patients who had chronic blood pressure problems that had a sudden improvement once unprocessed sea salt was introduced restoring completely normal pressure levels.

Nutrition's Playground

When Jesus said 'Ye are the salt of the earth' he was talking about this natural, life-giving, unprocessed salt that heals and supports the functioning of the human body. He was not speaking of the highly processed, imitation salt that unbalances and damages the systems of the body. Somehow we have come to accept this fraud as real salt. Real salt is necessary for life. Use it! But use the right type, natural, hand harvested, unprocessed sea salt.

Nutrition's Playground

Step 5: The Fundamental Fat Controversy

In the years since the government introduced national guidance on nutrition there is one piece of advice that has stood strong during all that time and has rarely been brought into question. This standard has been virtually forged in stone since 1977. It resonates in the halls of every diet group and serves as the foundation to the vast majority of weight management plans across the globe. This unwavering mantra is that fat should contribute only a nominal amount of calories to our daily diet. Fat is the enemy! It should be minimised at all costs! Fat makes you fat after all. It's a simple formula really, why complicate the matter? In a survey of over 107,000 Americans seeking weight loss the majority indicated that their sole approach to achieving their goal was the removal of fat from their diet! If you want to look a little bit deeper science has indicated that too much fat in the diet causes coronary heart disease (CHD), the biggest killer in the Western world. Statistics for 2006 show that cardiovascular diseases claimed over 831,000 lives in the US alone. In the United Kingdom almost 240,000 lives were claimed in the same year. Despite a reduction in the social acceptance of smoking, cigarettes are still the number one cause of coronary heart disease. The next biggest contributing factor is usually identified as being diet. The British Heart Foundations says:

'It is now universally recognised that a diet which is high in fat, particularly saturated fat, sodium and sugar and which is low in complex carbohydrates, fruit and vegetables, increases the risk of chronic diseases – particularly cardiovascular disease (CVD) and cancer.'

Nutrition's Playground

From almost every mainstream angle the answer to all our dietary problems is blamed squarely on excess fat. Could this single nutrient group really be responsible for all our health problems? Heart disease, cancer, diabetes, metabolic syndrome, asthma, allergies, hormonal imbalance, depression, gout and arthritis have all had some science implicate fats as a causative factor. Fats, particularly saturated fats, are present in so many foods eaten by man today. Beef, pork, lamb, venison, goat, rabbit, chicken, turkey, duck, goose, liver, kidney, trout, mackerel, herring, sardines, anchovies, salmon, fish eggs, milk, cheese, cream, butter, eggs, coconut products and many different types of nuts. These are all foods that have been eaten by man for many generations. If fats are really the problem and are causing so many diseases, why did medicine not observe this before the 1930's - 1940's when heart disease began to rapidly increase? This is simply what we have been conditioned to believe, that fats are the culprit in our decline of health. Of course, we should not question this as it is grounded in solid science... Isn't it

Shaky origins

The basis of our current dietary guidelines was developed over a number of years, the heart of which has been a reduction in fat intake. It is essential that we understand how we came to believe such advice and what was ignored along the way. Physiologist Ancel Keyes, of the University of Minnesota, first proposed the lipid hypothesis in his 1953 six countries study. This particular study was published in a lesser known scientific journal at the time because it was not a widely held view and many people opposed the hypothesis even after this study. In a nutshell this hypothesis promoted the idea that an increase in fat in the diet was associated with an increase in the number of coronary heart disease deaths.

Nutrition's Playground

Since that time there have been countless studies carried out looking at various aspects of this hypothesis. It has also developed to include the concept that elevated blood cholesterol is a significant factor in heart disease. In order to give this discussion its rightful place it is necessary to review some of the major events that have both contributed and challenged the lipid hypothesis. Despite the British Heart Foundation and many others claiming that the lipid hypothesis is 'universally' accepted there has always been a strong opposition that do not agree. If this is news to you then pay close attention and open your mind to the powerful counter arguments of the lipid hypothesis.

The first recorded event of someone dying of a heart attack in the US was in 1921. By 1930 there had been approximately 3000 recorded deaths. This growing trend soon led to further examination of this new problem. The earliest investigations into the idea of any type of fat causing CHD was shortly after the great depression in 1936. Two forensic scientists, Kurte Lande and Warren Sperry, investigated blood cholesterol levels and compared them to the level of fatty deposits found in the aorta, the first major artery leading blood away from the heart. Simply put, they found absolutely no correlation or trend between blood cholesterol and the level of blockage in any of the arteries of those who had suddenly died. This study seemed to have some influence as very little research was carried out in this area again until after the Second World War. By the time the Second World War had reached its end heart disease had become a rising problem in the US with the number of deaths from CHD peaking some years after in the 1960s. It has since held the title of the number one killer in the USA, and many other Western countries for that matter. Political, health and business interests were raised and research moved forward with new vigour in search for answers to this considerable problem.

Nutrition's Playground

After Ancel Keyes had published his research in the early fifties much more effort was made to direct the public in the kind of foods that should be eaten to prevent the development of heart disease. In 1956 the American Heart Association aired a television programme on all three major US networks as a fundraiser into research behind this dreaded disease. The panellists presented their views and ultimately promoted the change to a new eating regime they called the 'Prudent Diet.' This was an effort to encourage the public to replace butter, lard, beef and eggs with apparently 'healthy' alternatives such as corn oil, margarine, chicken and cold cereals. This would have proved a very successful programme except that not all of the experts on the panel were in agreement with what was being encouraged. Dr Paul Dudley White had been invited onto the show to offer his expert opinion.

Dr White was a highly respected cardiologist at the time. Two years after he first qualified as a doctor in 1911 he was offered the chance to go to London and study cardiovascular physiology, this was a decision that proved invaluable and changed the direction of his career. Several of his colleagues advised him against such a move suggesting he focus his efforts on an area of medicine with greater need. He first saw the electrocardiogram in England and brought it to the US in 1914 believing it would be invaluable in detecting early signs of heart irregularities. In 1924 he was one of the founders of the American Heart Association (AHA) and in 1941 Dr White became president of the AHA. Between 1921 and 1956 he worked as part of the Harvard Medical Faculty becoming an emeritus professor in 1949. He was the chief consultant to the National Heart Institute from 1948 to 1955 and was called upon to be President Eisenhower's physician following his heart attack in 1955. At the time of this AHA sponsored

Nutrition's Playground

television programme he was the president of the International Society of Cardiology.

Dr White was a man of considerable importance in the world of cardiology, and to the success of this programme. However, he did not completely agree with his fellow panellists on this television programme and boldly stated:

'See here, I began my practice as a cardiologist in 1921 and I never saw an MI (myocardial infarction / heart attack) patient until 1928. Back in the MI free days before 1920, the fats were butter and lard and I think we would benefit from the kind of diet that we had at a time when no one had ever heard of the word corn oil.'

Despite Dr White's expert opinion the stone had begun rolling and the lipid hypothesis was gaining momentum. In the year following this much talked about television programme Dr Norman Joliffe, a well respected expert in disease and nutrition and head of the Bureau of Nutrition in New York City's Department of Health, decided to put this eating regime to the test with an experiment he called the Anti-Coronary Club. He enlisted 814 men between the ages of 40 – 59 to serve as an experimental group that would eat a diet similar to the Prudent diet. Beef, mutton and pork were limited to 4 meals a week, poultry and fish were to be consumed at least 4 meals a week, butter and hydrogenated shortenings were replaced by polyunsaturated margarines and 1 ounce of vegetable oil each day, and finally ice cream and hard cheeses were avoided completely. 463 men were enlisted to serve as a control group to make comparison, though collected data for this group were taken much less often and dietary intake was not specified to ensure relevant opposites were achieved.

The study was published several years later in February 1966. The results clearly demonstrated that their dietary regime had lowered cholesterol significantly, whilst the control group had similar cholesterol as at the start of the trial. They also showed that the diet group had 8 new 'coronary events' and the control group had 12 new 'coronary events', a term which sounds like this was the number of heart attacks. This led to strong conclusions that their diet had proved beneficial and had a positive effect on heart disease risk. Upon further investigation the term 'coronary event' is defined by the authors to be one of 7 different categories from an actual heart attack to feelings of angina or chest pain. However, what is not discussed or factored into the results is that the control group had a much higher percentage of smokers than the diet group. It was also only briefly discussed that the diet group had a greater percentage of overweight subjects that were initially placed on a 1600 calorie weight loss diet until weight was normalised and then shifted over to the experimental diet. This was not carried out with the control group whose overweight subjects were left as they were; after all they were the control group. If you are really sharp when reading the article you would notice the number of fatalities that occurred during the study. First of all the fine print identifies that there were 8 deaths from heart disease in the diet group and none in the control group. There were also 18 non heart disease deaths in the diet group and only 6 in the control group. This shows that a total of 26 deaths from all causes occurred in the diet group whilst only 6 deaths occurred in the control group. So regardless of the decrease in plasma cholesterol the number of actual deaths was over 4 times higher in the Prudent diet group. Unfortunately Dr Norman Joliffe did not make it through the trials and died himself of a 'coronary event' in 1961.

This study was not honestly evaluated and added fuel to the growing fire that dietary intake when altered appropriately can lower the risk factors for heart disease. It also further suggested that cholesterol levels are linked with increased heart disease problems. This study was beneficial to the American Heart Association because it had put to the test their 'Prudent Diet' and published positive support for this approach. Yet the bottom line is that the study was flawed in its design and total death rate was underplayed in the results.

1958 was a significant year in the solidification of the lipid hypothesis because the first text book on cholesterol was published by Russian scientist, David Kritchevsky, simply titled 'Cholesterol'. This text referred to the data that cholesterol levels were elevated in individuals who had CHD and in those who had died of myocardial infarction.

This added a new element to the hypothesis, that is, both saturated fat content and cholesterol were now risk factors for heart disease because of their role in creating atherosclerosis in the arteries. With yin yang like balance, later the same year Laurie published a study in the globally respected medical journal, the Lancet, looking at the degree of atherosclerosis in various tribal groups in South Africa. He compared the virtually vegetarian Bantu tribe, with low saturated fat and cholesterol intake, to other tribes who had higher meat intakes and therefore higher saturated fat and cholesterol. He identified that the Bantu had remarkably similar levels of atherosclerosis as the meat eating groups despite the fact that their diet was considered to be more heart healthy at the time. Yet this study seemed to have little impact on the direction of the current scientific trend with regards to diet and heart disease.

In 1961 the AHA released its guidelines on dietary intake and lowering rates of heart disease and stroke. This was particularly interesting as there had not been any convincing evidence to date that changing the diet would have any positive influence on heart disease markers. This particular

Nutrition's Playground

point was backed up a few years later in 1969 when the Diet Heart Review Panel of the National Heart Institute (now National Heart Lung and Blood Institute) stated:

'It is not known whether dietary manipulation has any affect whatsoever on coronary heart disease.'

The 1961 AHA report was written by 4 men, one of whom was Ancel Keys and another called Jeremiah Stamler, a man who we will find out later has had quite an influence on our dietary views.

American Heart Association Report – 1961
1. Maintain a correct bodyweight
2. Engage in moderate exercise, e.g. walking to aid in weight reduction
3. Reduce intake of total fat, saturated fat, and cholesterol. Increase intake of polyunsaturated fat
4. Men with a strong family history of atherosclerosis should pay particular attention to diet modification
5. Dietary changes should be carried out under medical supervision

Two significant studies were published soon after, in 1968, that should have received much more attention than they actually did. The first was authored by Malholtra and published in the Indian Journal of Industrial Medicine. He determined that the natives of northern India consumed 17 times more saturated fat in their diet, but had a CHD rate 7 times lower than the people of southern India. Another clear sign that dietary intake may have had less of a role in CHD than was justifiable at the time.

The second study really should have been enthusiastically shouted 'from the rooftops' because of the sheer size and volume of the data collected. McGill published the results of The International Atherosclerosis Project in which 23,205 corpses across 17 nations were examined for levels of arterial plaque. Upon examination of the immense data it was found that average levels of atheroma were similar across all parts of the world. This trend was still present whether they had eaten plenty of fatty animal products or whether they were largely vegetarian. The same average trend was still present even when there were significant rates of heart disease within the population group or if they suffered very little at all.

Opportunity missed

Following a 1970 report from a study being performed in the town of Framingham, Massachusetts, which displayed a poor correlation between cholesterol levels and heart disease, it was decided something more substantial was needed to determine once and for all if there was a cholesterol link. In 1971 the National Institutes of Health (NIH) task force determined what it would take to run a trial with a large enough study group to obtain enough data for more conclusive evidence. The focus of such a trial was to investigate whether a low fat diet would actually increase life expectancy without posing too many risks. The cost of such a study was estimated at $1billion! This was far beyond anything the NIH were willing to invest, or anyone else for that matter. So rather than fund a trial that may actually conclude the debate around a low fat diet, the NIH backed away and provided funding for a series of other smaller studies that totalled only a third of that cost. Many of these studies were observations of population groups, diets, lifestyles and medications and were set to last in the region of 10 years.

In 1974 a study was published regarding the dietary habits of Americans between 1900 and 1972 and showed that the intake

Nutrition's Playground

of animal sourced fats had declined in the diet from 104 to 97 g/person/day whilst the intake of vegetable oils had increased from 21 to 60 g/person/day. Despite animal fats still representing the greater proportion of fat in the diet, by 1972 there had been a slight decreasing trend whilst the use of vegetable oils by this point had virtually tripled during the same time that heart disease had risen from a virtually unknown problem to becoming the number one killer in the USA. It must also be recognised that the level of animal fat intake in 1900 was slightly higher than 1972 and yet heart disease was considered an obscure specialism at the time. Providing this data is accurate it seems impossible that animal fat intake could be the cause of heart disease as it goes against the trend. Another study to go against the trend was the Tecumseh, Michigan study published in 1976. The researchers stated that:

'Cholesterol and triglyceride levels were unrelated to quality, quantity, or proportions of fat, carbohydrate, or protein consumed in the 24-hr recall period.'

Although this looked only at food intake over 24 hours it involved over 2000 men and women and reviewed the dietary components of 2706 foods following which every person in the study had their plasma cholesterol tested. This was a very important study at the time especially considering what was to follow later that year and in early 1977!

Government involvement

Enter into the national dietary scene the failed presidential candidate, Senator George McGovern. During the past 4 years Senator McGovern had been working on reducing malnutrition in American inner city districts. Now that this work was drying up McGovern turned his attention to the

Nutrition's Playground

nutritional status of the country and in late 1976 sat with his own selection of lawyers and politicians for 2 days of training and direction on nutrition and the state of the American nation. This instilled in him the desire to set dietary goals for the American public to reduce the death toll being inflicted by heart disease. McGovern tasked a labour reporter, Nick Mottern, to write up these goals and present them back to the committee. Mottern was certainly no science writer and had a limited grasp of the subject and so relied heavily on the advice of a Harvard School of Public Health Professor by the name of Mark Hegsted. It must be said that Hegsted was no slouch in the world of science at the time. He had been involved in a lot of forward thinking research, particularly in the area of cholesterol, lipids and heart disease. He was a self confessed extremist in this area. A question worth asking at this point is if you consult an individual with a background in the lipid hypothesis to help provide dietary guidelines for the nation what are you likely to get? You guessed it, national dietary guidelines with a strong emphasis on reducing fat intake to try and reduce heart disease. Of course this is fine providing there is scientific evidence to support such a stance and as yet there was nothing conclusive.

In early 1977 the McGovern Senate Select Committee published what they called the 'Dietary Goals for the United States.' This was done with some pomp and grandeur at a large press conference. Mark Hegsted reported that the general response did not go as well as planned saying:

'All hell broke loose...practically nobody was in favour of the McGovern recommendations.'

The McGovern report did actually acknowledge the lack of existing data to prove that a reduction in dietary fat would decrease blood cholesterol levels and therefore lead to a reduction in heart disease. A bizarre irony when providing national goals to lower heart disease risk! However, this was justified by suggesting that because fat has approximately 9 calories per gram and protein and carbohydrates account for only 4 calories per gram then lowering fats in the diet would help reduce weight by lowering caloric intake. This was the back-up hypothesis to cover the weak diet cholesterol stance taken by the committee to support heart disease reduction. It is important at this point to fully understand exactly what the goals proposed by the McGovern committee were.

1. Increase carbohydrate consumption to account for approximately 55-60% of energy intake
2. Reduce overall fat consumption from 40% to 30% of energy intake
3. Reduce saturated fat consumption to account for about 10% of total energy intake; and balance that with polyunsaturated and monounsaturated fat, which should account for 10% of energy intake each
4. Reduce cholesterol consumption to about 300mg/day
5. Reduce sugar consumption by about 40% to account for about 15% of total energy intake
6. Reduce salt consumption by about 50-85% to about 3g/day

These guidelines do not look too far away from what we are advised to eat today through government guidelines. There are some minor value differences but the same basic message makes up today's guidelines. So why then was there such a revolt against the suggested guidelines that McGovern tried to introduce.

It seemed for a time like the Dietary Goals for the United States were going to fade away as people began to turn their attention elsewhere. However, towards the end of 1977 a keen

Nutrition's Playground

food activist, and then assistant secretary within the US department of agriculture, Carol Tucker Foreman, saw what McGovern had been trying to do and chose to try and stabilise the faltering US dietary goals. She understood the plight of the general public who had to continue to eat and feed their children every day despite increases in disease and felt we had to make public policy right now, even if the scientists still remained in the midst of dietary debate with no solid answers. Carol sought from scientists the 'best sense of the data right now.' To try and find out what this advice would be she went to the group that created the now well recognised Recommended Daily Allowances, the National Academy of Sciences Food and Nutrition Board. The president of this group at the time was an expert on human and animal metabolism, Phillip Handler. He was not interested in endorsing the McGovern recommendations and referred to them as 'nonsense.' Foreman turned to the National Institutes of Health for advice and was told that the McGovern guidelines were much more of a political document than scientific. The director, Donald Fredrickson said 'we should let the crazies on the hill say what they wanted.' The American Medical Association, the National Heart, Lung and Blood Institute and renowned University of London cardiologist Sir John McMichael all raised their voices in opposition to the McGovern guidelines.

It was eventually agreed that the USDA in conjunction with the Surgeon General's office would draft some official guidelines that could be put forward as official policy. Interestingly we find that Carol Foreman hired Mark Hegsted to head up this effort. As a result in February of 1980 the USDA released the Dietary Guidelines for Americans which looked remarkably similar to the original McGovern committee guidelines. At almost the same time a well respected researcher from Rockefeller University ,Pete

Nutrition's Playground

Ahrens, wrote to the British scientific journal, the Lancet, stating

'It is absolutely certain that no one can reliably say whether a change in dietary regimens will have any effect whatsoever on the incidence of [coronary heart disease], nor in whom.'

Only a few years later the British government adopted something similar to the USDA guidelines in establishing their own public policy on food and nutrition in 1984. So despite the uncertainty regarding the role of diet in the pathology of cardiovascular and heart disease both governments began to direct the public to make the biggest 'en masse' shift ever in dietary intake. The intention to try and improve health across the nation was admirable, but if the guidelines being provided were based on a best guess then the chance of error was high as well and perhaps could even decrease health markers rather than improve them. An interesting irony to this section of the history is that in 1981 Mark Hegsted returned his attentions once again to his job at Harvard School of Public Health where he continued his research under the funding of Frito Lay, a large potato crisp manufacturer owned by Pepsi!

Research continues

A scientific review of 3 major cardiovascular studies was published in 1981, which made some interesting observations with regards to their findings to that point. They compared individuals who had experienced heart attack to those who had not to see if any significant differences or risk factors were apparent. Surprisingly there were no significant differences in dietary cholesterol, polyunsaturated vegetable oils or saturated fat intakes. They did identify a few clinically significant factors with the heart attack population groups showing greater calorie, carbohydrate and alcohol intakes. It is amazing that this information could be published regarding 3 of the most significant cardiovascular studies by that point in time and hardly make a dent in US nutritional policy. Even more concerning is that the UK government was in consultation over their own forthcoming nutritional policies and this did not cause a change in their own decisions and eventual outcome just a couple of years later.

The following year in 1982 the Chicago heart trials were published which found that a lack of education correlated with an increased risk of heart disease. No pattern was found with cholesterol or fat intakes. Towards the end of 1983 the Nutrition Guidelines for Health and Education were published in Great Britain and later adopted as public policy early the following year. These guidelines, like those in the USA were not simply accepted and did raise some dissenting voices. They also acknowledged a complete change in direction of previous nutritional advice in relation to weight control.

'The previous nutritional advice in the UK to limit the intake of all carbohydrates as a means of weight control now runs counter to current thinking.'

In 1984 three major heart trials were published during the review of the US dietary guidelines. The Puerto Rico heart health study found little evidence between diet and heart disease except that drinkers of whole milk had half the risk of high blood pressure compared to those who did not drink milk, suggesting a role for calcium in CHD. The Honolulu Heart programme did identify a link regarding cholesterol in the actual heart attack event, but said it was not a significant risk factor in cardiovascular disease. This study strongly linked smoking and glucose intolerance with heart disease.

118

Nutrition's Playground

This was a significant point as it was one of the first major research trials to show a connection between carbohydrate excesses and the development of diabetic tendencies with heart disease problems. The trial that ended up getting the most attention was one called the Lipid Research Clinical Trial. This was a drug trial testing the efficacy of a cholesterol lowering medication; it was not a dietary trial. The new drug did show a significant reduction in heart disease at the same time as lowering cholesterol. This caused the authors to conclude that a change of dietary habits to reduce dietary cholesterol and saturated fats would bring about the same benefits of lower blood cholesterol and therefore a reduction in heart disease. There is no way that this conclusion could be fairly made as this study had nothing to do with dietary observations. It was a drug trial, nothing else. Yet this outcome, despite all the other major studies that found little evidence for diet in the role of heart disease, was to become a major influencing factor in the turn of events to follow!

Consensical

Towards the end of 1984 the National Institutes of Health decided to hold a consensus conference to bring together all the evidence regarding diet and health and to determine suitable recommendations for guiding the medical community. 20 speakers presented over the conference, many of whom towed the line regarding the dietary guidelines. It is amazing that this was the case when just a few short years earlier so many notable people and institutions had spoken against the guidelines that were proposed. Perhaps the difference was that the guidelines had now become public policy? There were a few who spoke out against the current evidence during this conference highlighting the lack of scientific rationale in support of the low fat dogma. However, when the conference report was published it made no mention of any discord and that the decision to move forward with their recommendations was unanimously agreed. It seems strange that at great cost such a conference would be hosted if everyone was in agreement. After all, why hold a 'consensus' conference if there was already an overwhelming consensus. Perhaps the most important guidance that came out of this NIH conference was the level of blood cholesterol that was set to be the safe upper limit. This was decided to be the nice and neat figure of 200mg/dL. The human body does not work in figures; it is not interested in rounded, simple to remember markers. In the UK cholesterol is measured differently and once converted over this represents 5.2mmol/L. Perhaps this is more believable because it isn't the nice, round figure that it was based on from the US conference. The following year the revised US dietary guidelines were released and looked virtually identical to the original guidelines despite the considerable volume of research that had been published that showed little support for the diet heart theory.

The idea was conceived in 1983 to run a major study in China to investigate what they were eating because heart disease rates were so low. This began what was to be known as 'The China Study' which became vital support to the current dietary guidelines. Interestingly the study, led by Professor T. Colin Campbell, selected to observe and measure health in mostly rural Chinese regions. Many of these regions had fairly modest living conditions and so lived off the produce of the land. Little meat was consumed, which is common in poor areas. The animals are more valuable for supporting the community by helping till the farmland and providing small amounts of animal produce like dairy and eggs. Some areas of China with more wealth are known for eating greater amounts of meat, but these were not included in the first survey or the second. The results of the study supported the

Nutrition's Playground

use of a plant dominant diet with reduced levels of fat as a method of minimizing heart disease. It is also interesting to note that Professor Campbell was a vegetarian. This rings of great similarities to the McGovern committee who instigated vegetarian reporter Nick Mottern to write the forerunning goals to the US dietary guidelines. The study was also heavily funded by cancer institutions and charities who had already adopted the national dietary guidelines in both the US and the UK.

Shortly after this event the dietary guidelines received another blow, interestingly enough from Japan! It had been well known for a time that China and Japan had some of the lowest heart disease rates in the world and many thought we needed to emulate their eating patterns in order to improve our health and reduce the risk of cardiovascular disease. This led many researchers going to Japan and China (as discussed above) to review what they were doing and to collect health data. Dr David Jacobs, a professor of public health from the University of Minnesota did just that. He learned whilst there that Japanese doctors often encourage their patients to raise their cholesterol levels rather than reduce them. This came as a surprise as the Western world had only just set on the upper limit of 5.2mmol/L and were now encouraging many people to lower their cholesterol in an attempt to reduce heart disease rates. As Japan had such low CHD rates they were more concerned about the diseases that were prevalent in their own region, such as hemorrhagic stroke. It turns out that this type of stroke, a bleed or rupture in the brain, is associated with low cholesterol levels, not high. When Dr Jacobs investigated scientific data he had available to him he observed this same pattern and became concerned regarding the current cholesterol education in the West. This eventually led to another major conference, this time hosted by the National Heart, Lung and Blood Institute (NHLBI) in 1990.

Nutrition's Playground

The NHLBI conference drew on a vast amount of evidence, collated from more than 19 studies and 64,000 deaths. After reviewing the data they found that this same concerning pattern of increased hemorrhagic stroke at lower levels of cholesterol was indeed present and a host of other diagnoses as well. In trying to determine the risk of all types of death and not just CHD they created a health risk score that took all causes of death into account. This was then compared to overall cholesterol levels. The data for men showed that there was indeed a slight increase in risk with cholesterol levels above 6.2mmol/L, but it also showed that an even greater risk for men was found at cholesterol levels below 4.1mmol/L. Men with low cholesterol had a greater risk from cancer, respiratory disease, digestive disease, aggressive behaviour, depression and suicide. The even bigger surprise, if that didn't go against the grain enough, was that increasing cholesterol levels in women were associated with lower rates of disease and poor health. When all causes of death were included women seemed to be protected by increased cholesterol.

This was probably one of the most in-depth, significant investigations of its time into cholesterol and health. Despite this the 1990 dietary guidelines were reviewed and released and looked remarkably similar to those that had gone before in 1980 and 1985. In 1991 an eminent researcher who had been a part of the longest running study on heart disease, the Framingham Study, planned to run a conference on the diet/heart hypothesis with his advertising for the conference stating it 'was the greatest scam in the history of medicine.' Unfortunately for Dr George Mann his conference didn't have the impact he had hoped as many of those invited were scared off. Dr Mann reported

Nutrition's Playground

'Scientists who must go before review panels for their research funding know well that to speak out, to disagree with this false dogma of Diet/Heart, is a fatal error. They must comply or go unfunded. I could show a list of scientists who said to me, in effect, when I invited them to participate: 'I believe you are right, that the Diet/Heart hypothesis is wrong, but I cannot join you because that would jeopardize my perks and funding.' For me, that kind of hypocritical response separates the scientists from the operators — the men from the boys.'

By 1992 this information, alongside the NHLBI conference, had made little effect on the direction that the public were being advised. As a result Dr Stephen Hulley of the NHLBI published a statement regarding the need for reform. He called for a change in the direction of public policy with regard to cholesterol education.

'We are coming to realise that the resulting cardiovascular research, which represents the great majority of the effort so far, may not apply to women ... the findings call into question policies built over several decades on evidence that focused only on CHD as an outcome . . . it may be time to review national policies aimed at shifting the entire population distribution of blood cholesterol'

This same year the USDA produced its famous dietary food pyramid in an effort to make the guidelines even clearer to the general public.

In 1993 Harvard professor Walter Willett published a study pointing out that a type of manmade fat called a trans fatty acid was a significant factor in the cause of heart disease. This implicated margarines and partially hydrogenated oils that had been used for decades by processed food manufacturers. The newspapers reported heavily on this study as a result of the controversy it created as margarines had been touted as healthy for 25 years by this time.

123

Nutrition's Playground

Truthfully ignorant

In 1994 another important study was published that did not receive much attention and, to be honest, was considerably overlooked. Yet the study was published in the Lancet, the 'gold standard' of all medical journals. This was the same scientific journal that published Willett's work on trans fatty acids the previous year. Carl Felton's research involved atherosclerotic plaques that build up on the inside of artery walls. In order to correctly determine what made up these plaques, scientists had literally been removing the material from dead bodies after autopsy and testing the plaque to see what it was composed of. This was to take away any theory or guess work surrounding the type of fats that are deposited within the arterial wall. The diet/heart hypothesis had always promoted the idea that it was saturated fat and cholesterol that was responsible for a considerable majority of the arterial plaque. Felton determined that only 26% of the fat located in artery clogs was saturated and the remaining was unsaturated fats. The greater majority (64%) of the unsaturated fats were found to be polyunsaturated, the very type of fat that had been encouraged for their benefits to the heart and the cardiovascular system. Felton stated:

'These findings imply a direct influence of dietary polyunsaturated fatty acids on aortic plaque formation and suggest that current trends favouring increased intake of polyunsaturated fatty acids should be reconsidered.'

The same year Dr George Mann backed up the claim made previously regarding trans fatty acids. He too had seen considerable evidence that these manufactured fats had a significant part to play in the pathology of heart disease and arterial damage. European research in 1995 found that trans-fatty acids were also positively associated with increased rates of breast cancer as well. 1995 also saw the release of the 4th edition of the dietary guidelines with very little change compared to what had gone before. Some direction was offered on nutrition labelling information and the food guide pyramid was adopted as part of public policy. It seems almost unbelievable that with so much new scientific information being brought out, and with so many challenges to the diet/heart hypothesis that the guidance offered on nutrition would remain the same. Yet the momentum that had now been built up through government and public departments continued to drive the same guidance that had been generated in the 1970's on an increasingly shaky foundation.

In 1998, following a nutrition conference that was focused on the nutritional value of dietary fat, Dr David Kritchevsky, the now retired author of the 1958 textbook on cholesterol, published a brief article. In this article he discussed some of the issues surrounding dietary fat and the current theory surrounding heart disease. Now, remember, this man had been a key part in laying those initial foundations implicating cholesterol and saturated fats as the culprits behind rising heart disease. Yet in this article he made a statement that was almost a complete reversal of his long held ideas. He said that the cause of coronary heart disease was not:

'as cut and dried as it may have appeared only a few short years ago'

Regarding the role of diet and drugs and their effects in scientific trials, he said that more recent evidence suggested they 'did not affect overall CHD mortality'. Respected scientists, even those like Kritchevsky and Mann who were involved in early research that helped form the dietary guidelines, were beginning to turn their backs on the lipid hypothesis due to the lack of valid supporting evidence.

Nutrition's Playground

Heart stats

In the same year that Kritchevsky stated that diet and drugs did not affect CHD mortality a revealing 10-year study came to its conclusion and was published in the New England Journal of Medicine. In this study they discussed the steadying and decrease in heart disease death rates in the US. This decrease in deaths from 502/100,000 in 1970 to 240/100,000 by 2002 is often used as 'proof' that the dietary guidelines, which were centred on reducing heart disease, have been working and improving national health. This study suggested that heart disease deaths had dropped as a result of improvements in medicine and that doctors were treating the disease more successfully rather than there being an actual decline in the occurrence. This is backed up with statistics produced by the American Heart Association. In 1979 they identified that there were 1.2 million medical procedures performed in the management of heart disease. However, by 1996 this number had rocketed to 5.4 million procedures. It appears that there were fewer heart disease deaths because so many more people were having their lives extended through surgery. Although it is to be commended that so many lives were saved during those years by modern medical intervention, it is shocking that it took millions of heart disease procedures combined with population wide dietary change at costs running into many billions of dollars to be able to observe this reduction in the heart disease mortality curve. How long can these difficult and costly interventions be sustained, before the increasing numbers of heart disease cases blow the lid off medical management capabilities?

In 1999 a study was published that finally had enough shock value to make a small alteration in public dietary advice. This publication was called the Lyon Diet Heart Study. This was a dietary study that put to the test a moderate fat, vegetable

126

Nutrition's Playground

rich diet called the Mediterranean diet and compared it to the AHA Prudent diet that was first conjured up in the 1950s. You may remember that the Prudent diet was previously tested in the 1960s by Dr Norman Joliffe and was trumped up to be a great success because it lowered blood cholesterol levels. Unfortunately more people died on the low fat Prudent diet than on the standard meat and potatoes diet. What made the Lyon study so unique was that it involved 605 heart attack survivors! The group was split in half and each group was observed over a period of 4 years. The impact to the scientific world came because at the end of the 4 years only 14 people had died in the higher fat Mediterranean diet whilst 44 had died on the low fat Prudent diet. With a death rate 3 times higher in the Prudent group this drew the attention of the scientific community and investigations were made as to why this higher fat diet seemed to be protective of the cardiovascular system.

The answer that has come to light since that time is that the Mediterranean diet is high in monounsaturated fats which have been shown to be beneficial to the arteries by keeping them free of plaque build up. It is also high in fresh, local vegetables rich in many protective vitamins, minerals and antioxidants. Mediterranean countries certainly exhibit lower rates of heart disease, but this does not protect them from gaining weight. Figures from the WHO's largest ever study on heart disease mortality, called MONICA (2000), show that the average level of overweight in Italy to be virtually identical to the UK at a body mass index of 26.4 and 26.3 respectively. However, Italy experience less than half the rate of coronary heart disease deaths compared to the UK. This is another clear sign that the dietary guidelines were being steered by one thing only – reducing the prevalence of heart disease mortality, not in minimising the rates of obesity, a potential heart disease risk factor.

Nutrition's Playground

A long awaited tweak

The 2000 edition of the dietary guidelines were released with a fundamental change. The guidelines stated that people should 'Choose a diet that is low in saturated fat and cholesterol (no change there) and moderate in total fat.' This was to create an allowance for increased monounsaturated fats in the diet to provide the protective heart benefits observed in the Lyon study. Another change was found in this edition. They also distinguished between refined and whole grain products encouraging people to emphasise the whole. This seems unusual as the Mediterranean diet was much richer in vegetables, but the emphasis here comes from grain products. There was one slightly confusing and contradictory point. The public were still being encouraged to be guided by the 1992 food pyramid. The pyramid at this point still said to eat fat sparingly and there was little distinction between whole and refined grain products in the illustration. These changes were not introduced to the pyramid until the 2005 edition of the national dietary guidelines. So for 5 years the national food guidance was contradicting itself. Another vital point to recognise here is not just that the governments finally recognised the strength of evidence from nutritional science, but that by changing their guidelines in 2000 and solidifying them in 2005 they in essence were admitting their previous guidance was wrong! No public apology, no embarrassment observed or even any mention of this was offered. For 20 years in the US and the UK and perhaps in many countries across the world, the national food policy had been telling people to lower their fat content to very low levels, with little supporting evidence that this actually lowered heart disease deaths, only evidence that it reduced cholesterol levels. How many deaths had been caused or how many people had their poor health

Nutrition's Playground

exacerbated as a result of this incorrect guidance remains to be determined.

It took 20 years of rigorous science to bring about some small amendments in the dietary guidelines. 20 years of less than optimal advice. It wasn't insufficient evidence that had prevented change either, just that the policy makers continued to ignore or keep up to date with the science that had been done. By now acknowledging that a change in national guidelines was necessary and that change was needed it can only raise questions about whether the current guidelines are going to fare any better. Will changes be applied in the future? Despite the apparent reduction in heart disease deaths since the introduction of dietary guidelines, the complete opposite is true of national obesity rates. According the US national NHANES surveys between 1960 and 1980 obesity rates rose from 12 – 15%, whilst after the introduction in national dietary guidelines in 1980 obesity rates had risen to 31% in 2000. According to UK national statistics obesity rates averaged 7% in 1980 and by 2001 they had risen to 21% in males and 24% in females. Have we just traded one health problem for another, a modest reduction in heart disease deaths for a doubling and tripling of obesity rates? It seems ironic that pointing the finger at dietary fat has resulted in massive increases in stored body fat and obesity rates. Perhaps the real problem is that national programmes have been trying to provide dietary advice to suit the mass population, a one size fits all approach.

Nutrition's Playground

Walter talks

In 2004 Harvard professor, Walter Willett, was interviewed on PBS television in a programme called Diet Wars. Dr Willett is one of the most cited scientists in all of clinical medicine and considered by some to be the world's leading nutritionist. So if anyone could provide some direction on dietary advice he would be a pretty safe bet. The national dietary guidelines were discussed and Dr Willett highlighted the significant effect they had imposed on the nation. Public policy directs everything from food production to supermarket stocking to educational programmes. Dr Willett was very honest admitting that he had advised patients poorly in his early years as a result of national guidance.

'Unfortunately, as a physician back in the 1980s, I was telling people that they should replace butter with margarine because it was cholesterol free, and professional organizations like the American Heart Association were telling us as physicians that we should be promoting this. In reality, there was never any evidence that these margarines, that were high in trans fat, were any better than butter, and as it turned out, they were actually far worse than butter.'

Willett, prior to this, had become a huge voice in the battle against manufactured trans fatty acids in the food supply, found in margarines and any foods containing partially hydrogenated vegetable oils. Willett also went on to discuss how the national dietary guidelines were not appropriate for the many overweight and obese people in the country because they were too high in starchy carbohydrates that shift their internal hormonal controls towards fat storage. Despite the recent changes in the dietary guidelines Willett still believed that they were not ideal for many in the population.

Nutrition's Playground

Women speak out

In 2006 the results of a 15 year research effort called the Women's Health Initiative (WHI) Dietary Modification trial were published. The WHI was one of the greatest undertakings in scientific history and involved over 161,000 women and cost many hundreds of millions of dollars. There were three major components to this trial, one of which was the dietary modification element. This set out to study the long term benefits of a low fat, high fruit, vegetable and grain based diet on 48,835 women. This was the largest dietary intervention study ever performed. The participants were followed every 6 months for a period of 8 – 12 years. The study group were taught 18 times about diet and nutrition within the first year and then attended 4 meetings a year lead by registered dieticians and nutritionists. This provided needed motivation and accountability to keep the study group on target. The objective was for them to eat only 20% of their calories from fat, at least 5 fruit and vegetables a day and at least 6 servings of grains a day. By the end of the 8.1 years of intervention the diet group had reduced their fat intake to 24-29% of total calories, had averaged slightly more than 5 portions of fruit and vegetables per day, but struggled slightly with grains to achieve just over 5 portions per day. This still differed

significantly from the control group who averaged over 35-37% of calories from fat, only 3 – 4 servings of fruit and vegetables and 4 servings of grain. The study was able to show the following results when the dietary change group were compared to the control group.

Breast Cancer
Control – 45 per 10,000
Diet – 42 per 10,000

Nutrition's Playground

Colorectal Cancer
Control – 12 per 10,000
Diet – 13 per 10,000

Cardiovascular disease
Control – 36 per 10,000
Diet – 35 per 10,000

It was also found that after nearly 9 years of intervention that the diet group had eaten approximately 300 calories less per day and maintained an average decrease in body weight of only 0.5 kg! Imagine that? 9 years of trying to eat healthier, being coached by dieticians, actually keeping fat intake down by 8-11% and still barely half a kilogram difference in body weight. How frustrating that must have been for the participants who stuck to their guns and kept up with the regime. Then to add to it no improvement in colorectal cancer at all and changes in breast cancer, heart attack and stroke were so small as to be clinically insignificant. Have you ever heard of the WHI Dietary Modification Trial before? It is the largest study of its kind ever performed in the world. Well, what would you do if you had spent hundreds of millions of public money on a trial that didn't come close to proving the long held theory that a low fat diet is necessary for health? Exactly, you'd keep it quiet!

In September 2007 the UK Food Standards Agency choose to revise their healthy eating guidelines to try and make the advice a little clearer for the general public. They released what is called 'The Eatwell Plate.' It is an illustration of a plate showing that a third of food should come from potatoes, grains and grain products, another third from fruits and vegetables and the remaining third split between meats, fish eggs, dairy and high fat, high sugar foods. Although certain

Nutrition's Playground

clarifications have been made to the guidelines over the years, the resulting advice looks very similar to what was first proposed by the American Heart Association way back in 1961and what was later proposed in 1977 by Senator George McGovern's committee, despite minimal evidence at the time to truly support such advice. Has this dietary advice been vindicated today and proven to be best for all?

The answer to this question can only really be answered if we understand what the purpose of dietary guidelines was in the first place. These guidelines were put in place primarily to deal with cardiovascular disease. Since the 1960s it has been the number one killer in many industrial countries and the guidelines, driven to lower fat, cholesterol and salt were all about reducing heart disease risk factors. They were not designed to reduce obesity as it was not a major problem at their inception. Neither were they designed to tackle any other chronic health problems. However, it seems today that these dietary guidelines form the backbone of nutritional advice no matter what health problems you have. If you are overweight, follow the national dietary guidelines. If you have cancer, follow the national dietary guidelines. If you have diabetes, follow the national dietary guidelines. If you suffer from any modern chronic disease whether it be asthma, eczema, arthritis, irritable bowel syndrome, diverticulitis, menstrual irregularities, infertility or many other conditions the adjustments regarding diet so often point us towards the universal answer of following the national dietary guidelines. Was it just fortunate that guidelines set up to tackle cardiovascular disease happened to provide benefit across so many chronic conditions? Has the number one cause of death, heart disease, become so much the focus of medical and health advice that it is now seen as unethical to provide any nutritional guidance that is not in keeping with these principles for fear of increasing CHD risk?

Nutrition's Playground

Trying to investigate the dietary needs of each one of these conditions would require substantial time and space and is not the purpose of this book. However, it would be beneficial to know if the national dietary guidance stood up under scrutiny in providing benefit for those who are at risk of heart disease. After all this is the very purpose for which they were created.

Modern admission

On the 9th November 2008 Pam Belluck published an article in the New York Times following the presentation of new findings regarding the leading cholesterol lowering drugs at an American Heart Association conference. The major findings within the JUPITER study were that statins had been found to lower the levels of a protein, called C-reactive protein, a significant influencing factor in the inflammatory process involved in heart disease. This was hailed as such a significant finding that may provide benefit to millions. Amidst all these grand life saving statements a small paragraph was printed that could have easily gone unnoticed.

'Scientists said the research could provide clues on how to address a long confounding statistic: that half of heart attacks and strokes occur in people without high cholesterol.'

It may come as news that half of all heart attack and stroke victims do not have high cholesterol. Yet the major focus of modern medicine is to lower blood cholesterol through a combination of diet, lifestyle change and medication. It is interesting to note that this is not new to the scientists, but is a 'long confounding statistic.' It has always been known that elevated cholesterol was not always present in those who suffered cardiovascular disease. Now there is another reason to medicate even more people with statins. If they do not

134

Nutrition's Playground

have the classic sign of increased cholesterol, but show other heart disease risk markers, this multifaceted medication has the ability to reduce inflammation and C-reactive protein too. The benefit was reported as almost a 50% reduction in risk. Yet the actual figures showed the difference between the medicated group and the control group to only be 0.9%. How could such a groundbreaking study create such contradictory results? This is because they used a risk score called relative risk.

Relative risk is a clever way of creating figures that have greater impact in studies where the actual incidence of a disease outcome is very low. Rather than looking at what the risk is solely within a single population group they compare the risks between different population groups. If one person out of a thousand was at risk of heart disease in a population and two out of a thousand at risk in another then the absolute difference in risk is that 1 more person out of every thousand will suffer from heart disease, a figure of 0.001%. However, if we were to report that in relative risk it would be viewed as a 100% increase in risk because 2 people in one population are twice the value of 1 in another population. The size of the population group is ignored and all focus is placed upon those who actually suffer from the disease.

The JUPITER study divided 17,802 people with cholesterol levels lower than 3.4mmol/L into two groups. In slightly less than two years the control group had experienced 251 primary events whilst the statin group had only experienced 151 primary events. This accounted for 1.8% of the population in the control group and 0.9% in the statin group. Because the statin group had half of the absolute risk as the control group (0.9 is half of 1.8) this is reported as a 50% reduction in risk and sounds mightily impressive. The reality is we are talking about a difference of 100 fewer people out of a total 8901 people that constituted the medicated group. Whilst this has made a difference to the 100 people not experiencing heart disease the figures are not nearly as significant as the reports make out. Often in medical science when groups are compared in clinical trials they report their findings by comparing one group to the other in relative risk rather than discussing the absolute risk figures.

Population wide proof

When population wide surveys have been made regarding fat intake and heart disease rates the confusion surrounding the dietary guidance that we have been provided continues. Rather than bring up all of these population surveys it would be prudent to focus on the largest ever heart disease risk study carried out to date, the World Health Organisation's MONICA study. This was performed across 38 population groups in 21 countries and 4 continents around the globe. 69,251 males and 69,187 females were surveyed across a ten year period of time. This was a study of monumental proportions and cost many millions of dollars, in fact some reports claim it to be the most expensive cardiovascular risk study performed to date. I want to impress upon you the sheer magnitude of this research project. Surely if there was a link to the level of fat intake in the diet and the risk of heart disease this immense study would have identified a clear association?

The data published after the completion of the study did show some indicators that certain trends in risk factors were occurring, such as a general increase in BMI indicating the population was becoming heavier, but interestingly a general decrease in cholesterol was also observed. When looking at actual figures the association between heart disease events, total fat intake and saturated fat intake does not show the

Nutrition's Playground

clear cut pattern that we have been taught to believe. The following table is adapted from figures published on www.heartstats.org from MONICA data and another WHO division called the Food and Agricultural Association (FAO). The data shown is for male events as they experience considerably higher rates of heart disease than females, in some areas even 3-4 times the rate.

Country	Average Coronary Events (per 100,000)	% Total Fat Intake	% Saturated Fat Intake	% Cholesterol above 6.5mmol/L
U.K.	736	35.1	13.5	31
Finland	701	36.2	14.4	36
Poland	524	29.8	10.7	22
Denmark	517	35.5	12.6	30
Lithuania	498	27.9	7.7	31
Iceland	486	36.2	14.6	36
Russia	470	24.7	8.3	10.5
Sweden	436	35.5	12.8	35.5
Belgium	416	40.3	14.5	37.5
Germany	339	36.7	14.4	32.5
France	274	41.8	15.5	36
Italy	266	38.2	11.8	28
Switzerland	261	40.1	15.3	47.5
Spain	210	41.2	10.9	21

Adapted from WHO MONICA study 2003

When looking at this data that has been gathered by the World's most respected health organisation it is astounding how we can draw the conclusion that fat intake or even saturated fat intake is linked to heart disease. The same

Nutrition's Playground

information has been plotted on a graph the country with the highest number of coronary events on the left and the lowest on the right.

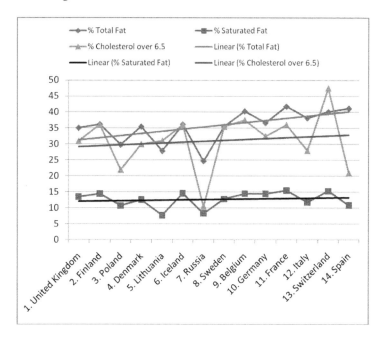

Adapted from WHO MONICA study 2003

Firstly we can see that there is no direct correlation between either total fat intake or saturated fat intake or the percentage of the population with cholesterol over 6.5 mmol/L and heart disease occurrence. There are some general trends shown by the additional trend lines. This shows that total fat and saturated fat generally increase as we move from left to right. Cholesterol levels also rise as the graph moves towards the right. Remember that the United Kingdom has the highest number of coronary events decreasing across the countries to the right to Spain which has the lowest. So if anything this

Nutrition's Playground

information shows that there are fewer coronary heart problems in countries eating more total fat and more saturated fat with higher cholesterol levels! To add to this Poland, Lithuania and Russia have the lowest total fat and saturated fat intakes across the group and they are all in the left half of the chart with higher heart disease rates. Poland and Russia also have very low cholesterol levels. Although this information does not suggest a cause for the increasing or decreasing heart disease rates, it is clear that fat intake, whether total or saturated, and cholesterol levels are not the cause of coronary heart disease when looking at the largest ever study on heart disease risk in conjunction with official FAO fat intakes of the same time period.

During the formation of national dietary guidelines there was plenty of evidence that seems to have been overlooked that suggested that dietary fat and cholesterol was not the only factor involved in the increase in heart disease. If anything some data suggested that certain fats were protective against hearts disease. Monounsaturated fats like olive oil and the essential omega 3 fats have been shown to be protective and this is now well accepted in mainstream science. However, the attack on saturated fats continues despite a significant amount of evidence suggesting that at worst saturated fats are neutral when it comes to heart disease. Why would we evolve to eat foods rich in saturated fats if it was so detrimental to our health? Many of the foods so rich in these fats have been part of indigenous diets for many centuries without the damaging effects of modern chronic diseases. Modern science, government, food marketing and other propaganda have created a world of fat phobics who are trying desperately to be healthy in order to enjoy life to the full. This is unnecessary and may even be detrimental to their health.

Nutrition's Playground

Fat in all its naturally occurring forms is an essential nutrient that should be part of our daily diet. It is manmade hydrogenated and trans fats and many readily available polyunsaturated oils, that have become rancid through processing, that should be avoided. It is man's interference through manufacturing and processing the fats in our food that is causing the problems! So who stands to gain from the propagation of these mistruths? Perhaps the most obvious is the vegetable oil industry itself! By radically changing population wide beliefs they have generated a vast market for their highly processed oils, margarines and low fats spreads. They market directly to consumers and to the processed food industry claiming they offer the answer to meeting national food guidance for lowering saturated fat intake.

Soya bean oil is the most commonly used vegetable oil closely followed by rapeseed. Soya bean oil accounted for 59% of global oilseed production in early 2010 with production expected to rise to 307 million tonnes by 2020. This is worth staggering amounts of money across global markets. The November 2009 price for soya bean oil was $854 per metric tonne making the value of this volume of oil at these prices an unbelievable $262 billion! Corporations are generating astounding levels of wealth on the belief that we should eat less saturated fat by emphasising vegetable oils.

What price has been paid within the population for the accumulation of this extreme wealth? Perhaps the ultimate price has been the health of the many populations around the globe as we have witnessed vast increases in cardiovascular disease and obesity since the introduction of these cheap, processed oils into the food supply.

The following table details many sources of fats and oils and their fatty acid composition. This will serve as a fundamental resource in understanding what types of fat are contained

Nutrition's Playground

within the different food sources so that you can choose as an informed consumer.

All figures are derived from Know Your Fats by Dr Mary Enig PhD.

Nutrition's Playground

Source of Fat or Oil	Saturated	Mono	Poly	Ω 3	Ω 6
Coconut oil	91% (63% MCT)	6%	3%		
Palm Kernel oil	84% (54% MCT)	14%	2%		
Butter	66% (7% SCT, 5% MCT)	30%	4%	1%	3%
Cocoa butter	60%	38%	2%		
Lamb tallow	54%	35%	5%		5%
Beef Dripping	49-54%	42-48%	3-4%		3%
Palm oil	49%	40%	10%		9%
Human milk fat	48% (18% MCT)	33%	16%		
Lard	44%	45%	11%		11%
Duck fat	35%	50%	15%		14%
Chicken fat	30-32%	48-50%	18-23%		
Goose fat	29%	59%	11%		11%
Turkey fat	29%	44%	23%		23%
Cottonseed oil	29%	18%	52%		52%
Peanut oil	22%	46%	31%		31%
Avocado oil	22%	60%	18%	1%	17%
Cod liver oil	21%	57%	20%	15%	1%
Olive oil	15%	73%	10%	>1%	9-10%
Soybean oil	15%	22%	62%		61%
Sesame oil	15%	41%	43%		43%
Corn oil	14%	27%	59%	1%	57%
Sunflower oil	13%	18%	69%		69%
Grapeseed oil	11%	16%	73%	1%	72%
Flaxseed oil	9%	17%	74%	60%	14%
Walnut oil	9%	23%	66%	12%	54%
Evening Primrose oil	9%	9%	82%		82%
Safflower oil	8%	13%	78%		78%
Hemp seed oil	8%	12%	78%	19%	59%
Canola oil (LEAR)	6%	56-66%	29-36%	10%	19-26%
Rapeseed oil	4%	16%	80%	10%	14%

Nutrition's Playground

Step 6: Modern Myths and Misunderstandings

Food science and technology has introduced to us many hundreds and thousands of new food products that were not available to eat or buy only a few decades ago. Today many of us know no differently as we have had these foods available for the whole of our lives. They have become so common place that many would not even question whether these foods have nutritional value or are harmful because they have become ingrained into life and routine. To question their benefit would possibly lead to reasons for their reduction or avoidance in the diet. Therefore, it is easier to remain uninformed so that enjoyable habits and dietary intake can remain the same. I am assuming that you are reading this book because you want to be informed; you want to know about the benefits and dangers of the food that influence us. This chapter is going to discuss these new foods and also several myths that have built up over the years, some even reaching a level of dogma. Challenging these long founded beliefs regarding food and diet is often frowned upon as extremism. You decide.

Counting calories

The idea that national and global problems associated with our ever increasing waistlines are a direct result of the energy unit called a calorie has pervaded society's thoughts and beliefs almost to saturation point. Endless television shows, doctors, scientists, nutritionists and personal trainers preach the logic that losing weight is all about burning off more than we take in. This is almost always met with complete agreement as everybody acknowledges this dogmatic statement. Is the answer to the obesity epidemic really as simple as that? How come there was very little overweight and obesity before the general public really knew what a calorie was, yet now that it has become part of everyday language we struggle to keep the pounds off? It seems the more we focus on counting calories the more we attract the excesses of life on our hips, thighs and bellies.

What we typically call a calorie is actually a kilocalorie. This is the amount of energy it would take to heat 1 litre of water a single degree celsius. Food calories are measured by placing a sample of food into a testing device called a bomb calorimeter and literally exploding it within a sealed system and measuring the energy given off in the form of heat. There are specific values provided for the different food types but normally, to avoid confusion, it is simplified to be 4 kcals of energy for each gram of carbohydrate or protein based food and about 9 kcals for a gram of fat. This gross over simplification has led many on the diet trail to leave fat out of their food because, obviously, it carries the highest amount of calories per gram and has the most potent effect on lowering total energy intake. The added incentive to remove fat because it has been linked to heart disease problems has certainly served to strengthen the case for its reduction when trying to lose weight.

The majority of people keep an eye on their calorie intake by reading the numeric data printed on the outer packaging of many food products, in particular the nutrition table that is often present. The Foods Standards Agency ran a study of over 700 food products in relation to the accuracy of the values stated on the labels. They found that only 7% of the foods they tested actually met the stated values listed on the

Nutrition's Playground

labels! The law allows for natural variability of food and so provides a 20% leeway of values above or below that stated on the label. While many foods tested did contain levels within this range, nearly 25% of the foods tested had values that exceeded the generous 20% leeway. So the next time you pick up a cereal bar for a healthy snack that states it only contains 100kcals, know that these 'typical values' have a 1 in 4 chance of containing over 120 calories! This considerably decreases the chances of accurately counting your calories. 93% of packaged foods do not state the exact measure of calories correctly on the food label or the nutritional values table.

We are always told that excess energy will be stored as body fat and contribute to weight gain. Whilst this statement is true we have to seriously consider how we quantify what 'excess' is from person to person. Typical guidelines state that males should take in 2500 kcals per day and females' 2000 kcals per day. These are primarily used because they are simple and amounts that many people can easily remember. Neat figures always need to be questioned. The actual amounts in the national guidelines are 2550 kcals for men and 1950 kcals for women. These are still nice rounded figures. The human body doesn't care about the 'niceness' of the mathematics. It is governed by the nerves, hormones and metabolism and none of them consults the calculator before making a decision, so why should we? Perhaps you have come across charts or equations that provide more accurate estimates of calorie needs based on body weight, gender, height and activity levels. Equations for determining daily energy needs are often used to provide a more accurate estimate. The different variables taken into account are definitely valuable factors that will alter daily needs, but once again it only provides an estimate. It is feasible to have two different men both 30 years old, moderately active, 6 foot tall and 100 kilograms, but one have 30% body fat and the other only 15% body fat. This would suggest that one had 15kg of lean tissue more than the other. Lean tissue is generally considered to be more metabolically active than body fat tissue. There is no way that they both have the same energy needs, yet even these more reliable equations and calorie estimates will calculate their daily needs as being the same.

Physics and food intake

The 'calories-in versus calories-out' dogma has its roots in a law from the physical sciences, the first law of thermodynamics. This law basically states that when heating a system the total change in heat is determined by the total heat added to the system minus any heat lost from the system. This makes perfect sense. If we were to boil a kettle to reach 100 degrees Celsius, enough energy would need to be transferred into the water by the heating element to reach this temperature. However, there would also be heat lost into the air from the escaping steam and through convection to the surroundings. When you apply this logic to the human body it implies that we work just like a machine or simple heating system. What you eat minus what you excrete and burn off will total the energy applied to the human body. If this is in excess you will gain weight and if this is lacking you will lose weight. If it was really that simple surely we would have grasped it by now and there would be no problem with overweight and obesity! The equation that is used when discussing energy balance is as follows:

Change in body weight = food eaten – energy burned

This may seem familiar. It forms the basis of most calorie restricted diets and weight loss exercise programmes. But there is a fatal flaw in this equation, based upon an

Nutrition's Playground

assumption that is usually made. The assumption is to do with the direction of the equation, the causality. We always assume that the change in body weight is the outcome. If we eat too much and live a sedentary life we will put on weight. Whilst these indeed are factors to consider it is not the only way to look at this energy balance equation. The equals sign only indicates that the figures on either side must balance or be the same. Consider these simple equations:

$$6 + 4 = 10 \qquad 10 = 6 + 4$$

It does not matter which way we write the equation both are correct and balanced on either side of the equals sign. 10 is not the cause of 6 + 4, neither is 6 + 4 the cause of 10. If we apply this same mathematical truth to the energy balance equation we cannot assume that it only works in one direction, namely, that a change in weight is the result of too much food and too little activity. Mathematical law allows the equation to work in the opposite direction too. This then suggests that an increase in body weight may well be the cause of less activity and eating more food. This is just as plausible as the first option no matter how unusual it may seem. Think about anybody you know who is overweight. How would they describe their energy levels? I would bet that in most cases they would feel tired, fatigued or lacking in energy. This is a little unusual as the very nature of being overweight would suggest they have a significant excess of energy stored on their frame. Think of the last time you were tired, I mean really dog-tired. Did you go rushing off to the gym for a workout, or out on the street for a jog? I would imagine not and if you did it likely took great effort that ended up in a lack lustre exercise session. When you are tired and your energy levels are lacking, what might be your course of action to restore your flagging get up and go? It is probably one of two things, getting some needed sleep or getting something to eat. So here we have a perfectly sensible thought process that shows the equation can run the other direction. If we gain weight the extra load takes more energy to carry around leaving us lacking energy which in turn leads to less available energy for activity and exercise. The desire to rest and a need for food are natural responses to help us recover and hopefully give us a needed boost. Unfortunately neither rest nor more food will make the excess weight go away. Gaining weight can indeed be the cause of becoming lazy and eating too much!

Simply individual

Last of all we must ask what variations exist within each individual and what nutrient requirements they have from the food they eat. Over 80% of proteins eaten do not contribute towards daily energy, but are utilised for structure and function. A significant portion of the fats we eat also contribute to cell structure, nerve formation and hormonal controls. The amount of proteins and fats required will vary from person to person and in relation to individual levels of growth, stress, sleep, toxic load, work, rest, deficiency and general health. Levels of carbohydrate will also vary in accordance with biochemical individuality. Different digestive dysfunctions, many of them common, can affect the energy we receive as well. These can include hypoacidity in the stomach, liver dysfunction, gall bladder problems, pancreatic hypofunction, gut bacterial dysbiosis and variations from diarrhoea to constipation. Each of these diminish the quality of digestion and how much of the actual food eaten ends up digested and absorbed into the bloodstream. Just because we have eaten a food item does not mean that we are able to fully utilise it. The digestive tract is a hollow tube from entrance to exit and until the food is broken down and absorbed into the blood it is not useable by the body. If digestion is poor then food will pass through and out of the exit only partially digested. A 300 calorie meal does not mean that 300 calories are absorbed. Today with digestive distress being so common this situation is highly probable.

So where do you start? How do you count calories to use this theory of negative energy balance successfully for weight loss? Well that is the point, isn't it? It is virtually impossible, yet it is one of the most common methods used for weight management. No wonder the chances of success are so hit and miss. We even have a common term used for this lack of success in the English language because we have observed the failure of calorie counting so often - Yoyo dieting!

Small Regular Meals

Eating little and often is a strategy that has been used with increasing regularity as part of 'healthy' habits for weight loss. There are usually several reasons used for justifying eating little and often.

- To maintain a more consistent blood sugar throughout the day and reduce cravings and hunger

- To maintain more suitable insulin levels and so reduce the level of fat storage that occurs

- To increase metabolism and therefore add to potential weight loss

- To improve blood cholesterol levels

This grazing type approach usually involves at least three normal meals plus 2 snacks throughout the day, though this

Nutrition's Playground

has been taken to extremes and people have been encouraged to eat as many as 8-12 small meals a day in some diets.

Insulin is a hormone that is released from the pancreas after food intake to help direct tiny food particles that have been absorbed into the blood stream to travel into the cells around the body that need it. Insulin has its strongest response to carbohydrate intake closely followed by protein. It is very unlikely that fat would be the sole constituent of a meal, but if it was this would bring about almost no insulin response. Usually a meal will contain varying amounts of these major nutrients and therefore the insulin response will be stimulated by the composition of the meal and the amount taken in. As a general rule the more processed the meal, the greater the percentage of carbohydrate and the larger the meal actually is, the greater the insulin response will be. Modern dietary guidelines have encouraged us to shift our diets towards greater dependence on carbohydrate, with intakes of 50-60% of daily calories. Although food guidelines do not encourage this, the processed food industry has refined and marketed many cheap, carbohydrate based foods and snacks which are eaten with increasing regularity in modern cultures. White bread, pasta, white rice, pizza, chocolate, confectionery, crisps, fries, soft drinks and many other foods are laden with refined carbohydrates and as such will bring about a large and faster insulin response.

One of the problems with a fast, large insulin response is that blood sugar is sent to the cells much quicker than the insulin can be removed from the blood. This usually leads to a reaction where insulin pushes too much sugar out of the blood stream leaving levels too low for a period. This is called reactive hypoglycaemia. There are mechanisms to restore blood sugar when this happens, but it takes a little while for these to correct the situation. In the meantime the individual

150

Nutrition's Playground

will experience symptoms of hunger, cravings, fatigue, mental fog, poor concentration and in a severe hypoglycaemic incident even shakiness, slurred speech and loss of colour. Reactive hypoglycaemia will have been experienced by most people at some point. For others it is a regular occurrence mid morning or mid afternoon. This is often noticed by a dip in focus whilst at work and the need to perk up with a snack, tea, coffee or some other caffeinated drink. The most common quick food and beverages that people turn to in these desperate moments usually begin the whole reactive hypoglycaemia cycle again:

- a rapid rise in blood sugar
- a rapid rise in insulin to follow
- a rapid drop in blood sugar
- reactive hypoglycaemia
- a quick food or beverage is ingested

This reactive cycle is such a common feature in the daily life of the population it has almost become accepted as a perfectly normal part of modern living. It has been observed that hypoglycaemia is a time when food choices are often at their worst when cravings are strong and blood sugar needs to be restored. The advice to eat little and often is used as an antidote to this dilemma by arming people with the knowledge that they should eat regularly and to prepare in advance so they have healthy choices to hand to respond before hunger becomes too great. Whilst this is a better answer than falling prey to fatigue and intense cravings that lead to poor quality snacks, it still only deals with the symptoms of the problem rather than the root cause. This suggests that we can do nothing about the regular cravings that come along, but should bolster our blood sugar more often with food intake so the reaction is less severe. The question that needs to be looked into is why cravings are

Nutrition's Playground

becoming such a regular part of the 24 hour cycle. A sensible meal pattern of 2-3 meals a day has been part of human culture for many years. This has mostly been built around employment and working for a living. There is no reason why this should be insufficient in modern life. This was the normal meal frequency before obesity and overweight became a national or global concern.

Meal time satisfaction

A suitable breakfast should be able to provide sustenance and satisfaction until lunch time and the same from lunch until dinner. If you find you cannot last that long then the previous meal should be evaluated for its nutritional content. All macronutrients, carbohydrates, proteins and fats play a role in providing satisfaction and in keeping appetite at bay. Therefore all three should feature as a part of every meal. This sounds like a simple statement, but can change meal times considerably. Breakfast cereal, fruit or low fat yoghurt have too much carbohydrate and little protein or fat. A salad sandwich, fruit, crisps and a soft drink for lunch deliver the same high carbohydrate mix. The evening meal is often the only meal in the day where a greater portion of protein is eaten, often in the form of chicken, fish or other meat. This meal may still have a dominance of carbohydrate from larger servings of rice, pasta or potatoes. Although carbohydrates are satisfying and will quickly stimulate the production of gut hormones that communicate with the brain and decrease hunger, these particular gut hormones have a fairly short lived mechanism. This is why you may often feel like you need a 'top up' snack shortly after a carbohydrate dominant meal. We usually call this dessert! Proteins have been shown to provide the most significant down regulation of appetite and stimulation of satiety related gut peptides. Fats cause only minimal stimulation of gut peptides, but help

Nutrition's Playground

considerably between meals in maintaining energy levels and delaying the onset of future appetite and cravings.

The macronutrient content of a meal will also significantly affect the insulin response. Carbohydrate dominant meals, particularly from refined sources will bring about much larger insulin responses. Proteins stimulate insulin as well, but not as much as carbohydrate, whilst fats have little influence on insulin levels. As discussed, high insulin levels will lead to reactive hypoglycaemia. In trying to maintain more stable insulin and blood sugar levels it is important that those levels are maintained within appropriate ranges. Maintaining high blood sugar and insulin levels can be detrimental to health. Regular intake of carbohydrate dominant meals and snacks is a sure way to stimulate this scenario. Continually elevated levels of blood sugar and insulin over time will lead to impaired glucose tolerance, which will lead to weight gain and may eventually cause Type 2 diabetes. A healthy individual will feel energetic and alert providing blood sugar stays within the normal range. It is only when these levels drop too low that fatigue and poor concentration set in. However, there are very few outward symptoms to inform us that blood sugar is too high, except at extreme levels.

Eating a greater abundance of whole food carbohydrate sources together with suitable quality proteins and fats will maintain and balance blood sugar and insulin for longer periods throughout the day. It will be easier to sustain yourself from meal to meal with less need for snacks in between. It may take a little while to condition yourself to fewer meals per day if you have been eating little and often in this grazing approach. One of the hormones responsible for appetite, called ghrelin, is released from the stomach and signals to instigate sensations of hunger. This mechanism is influenced by routine and timing and can be synchronised with normal eating patterns. So when a change to meal times is introduced the ghrelin response still stimulates appetite at the previous habitual times for a short period until it learns the new routine that has been adopted. This can be challenging initially, but soon adjusts to match the new schedule.

Many studies have been performed and published within scientific literature on the topic of meal frequency. Comparisons have been made between as little as 2 meals to as many as 12 meals in one day. Some research has shown that there is no link to an increase in metabolism of those who eat twice a day and those who eat up to 7 meals per day providing the amount of food eaten is not different. It has also been shown that the amount of energy used in digestion is similar between 2 meals and as many as 12 meals a day, again providing the total energy input is the same. A single large meal does require more energy to digest, but this is offset by the longer time span between the 2 meals and so makes little difference. Research has also shown that smaller more regular meals have no influence on blood cholesterol levels. If total energy intake is kept the same smaller more regular meals has little influence on weight loss attempts. This is a strategy used to cover over the reactive hypoglycaemia brought on from meals and snacks with either lack of calories or too much carbohydrate.

Soured by sweeteners

The health risks associated with excess sugar intake have been known for some time. The message has permeated society to the point that an increasing market of low sugar or sugar free foods has grown in recent years. However, we have been gifted with the ability to taste sweet food and across all taste sensations the most preferred is sweetness.

Nutrition's Playground

This presents a dilemma. Too much sugar is bad for our health, but we like the taste of sweet food. Food manufacturers know that a loss of sweetness from a food product will decrease sales. The food industry has created an answer to this problem, artificial sweeteners.

The main no calorie or low calorie sweeteners on the market today are aspartame, sucralose, saccharin and acesulfame K. When sold purely as a sweetener they are usually branded and so may not be known by these names, but when added within processed food these are the names by which they are identified on the food label. Although their use does reduce the number of calories that would otherwise have been taken up by a sugar or syrup, it does not mean that they are a healthier option. Many who seek to lose weight do so to improve their image as well as their health. Artificial sweeteners are found in many diet foods, unsuspectingly increasing the risk of ill health amongst those who seek better health.

Aspartame is the most common artificial sweetener found in food today with estimates of it being used across more than 6000 different food products. It may be found in soft drinks, sugar free mints, sugar-free chewing gum, cocoa mixes, frozen desserts, jelly desserts, juices, milk shakes, yoghurts, laxatives, chewable vitamin supplements, pharmaceutical drugs and supplements, tabletop sweeteners, teas and instant coffee. Aspartame is approximately 200 times sweeter than table sugar. This intense sweetness means that only very small amounts need be used by manufacturers, which improves profit margins in comparison to using sugar. The taste of aspartame is not exactly like sugar and so it is often combined with acesulfame K to overcome this problem. Aspartame was discovered in 1965 by James Schlatter who worked for G D Searle and Company, but was not approved for use in dried foods until 1980 due to concern over studies

155

showing it caused cancer in rats. In 1983 its use was first broadened to include beverages and confectionery and then again in 1996 restrictions were removed completely allowing it to be used in any food product.

Controversy has surrounded aspartame ever since the first attempts to have it approved. Despite numerous statements from the US Food and Drug Administration that it is safe for human consumption within current allowable levels there are still many experts who warn against its use. Dr Russell Blaylock has campaigned against the use of aspartame for many years stating that it is an excitotoxin. After ingestion aspartame breaks down into its three component parts, 40% aspartic acid, 50% phenylalanine and 10% methanol. Methanol is converted into formaldehyde and then formic acid which is toxic to the body. Aspartic acid and phenylalanine are amino acids that are found in many foods. Aspartic acid is always bound together with other nutrients. Free aspartic acid, bound to nothing, is released into the body after aspartame ingestion. This amino acid in its free form crosses the blood brain barrier and stimulates neurons in the brain. These neurons can be excited so much that they shrivel and die, hence the name excitotoxin. Aspartame has been found to particularly damage the region of the brain known as the arcuate nucleus of the hypothalamus. This is the region of the brain responsible for monitoring appetite and the nutrients travelling in the blood supply. Therefore, aspartame has been shown to influence hunger levels and to have addictive qualities. This is clearly beneficial to the manufacturer who is trying to increase sales and profitability. Aspartame has been implicated as a contributing factor in Alzheimer's, Parkinson's, Huntington's, dementia, seizures, migraine, diabetes and meningitis.

Nutrition's Playground

Many have asked why the FDA or food governing bodies would allow a food additive into the food supply if it was considered to aggravate so many disease states. Research by Dr Ralph G Walton, a professor of clinical psychiatry, may shed some light on this. Dr Walton reviewed a scientific database called Medline for all the research he could find involving aspartame intake and human safety. At the time he identified 164 studies that met his criteria. 74 studies had aspartame industry funding whilst 90 studies had received funding from sources other than the aspartame industry. 83 out of the 90 studies (92%) with no financial incentive from the aspartame industry found there to be one or more safety concerns with the use of this sweetener. 6 of the 7 that did not identify a problem were run by the American FDA who had several staff that went to work for the aspartame industry immediately following its approval. Some consider these 6 studies to be influenced by pro-aspartame officials and as good as funded by the industry. All 74 of the aspartame funded studies claimed there to be no problems with regards to human safety and have given it a completely clean bill of health. There is a significant financial gain in aspartame having the 'safety' stamp of approval for the manufacturers of this toxic sweetener. Its current widespread use generates millions of dollars in revenue.

Sugar without the calories

Sucralose is a relatively new artificial sweetener and is being used with increasing regularity in modern processed food products. It is also beginning to replace aspartame as the sweetener of choice. This may be to keep consumers concerned about negative reports surrounding aspartame happy to still purchase food products which use sucralose, therefore maintaining sales figures. It may also be because sucralose is 600 times sweeter than sugar, making it 3 times sweeter than aspartame. This means that less can be used for the same relative sweetness and costs go down whilst profit margins increase. Sucralose is reported to be found in over 4000 food products and can be found in confectionery, soft drinks, cereal bars, protein shakes and in the low calorie sweetener branded as Splenda. Studies looking into sucralose safety and adverse side effects have shown it may contribute to shrinking of the thymus gland, reduced growth rate, and decreased red blood cell counts, losses in gut bacterial flora up to 50%, migraines and increases in body weight.

Sucralose is a chlorinated sugar that comes from the chlorocarbon family of chemicals. Officials have for many years taken the stance that sucralose is not absorbed by the body, but now indications show that approximately 15% of sucralose is absorbed, but they cannot guarantee which part! This means that when you add sucralose or eat a product with sucralose in it that you are gambling on your health. If we absorb the chlorine element from sucralose, then as with chlorinated drinking water, we are increasing our risk of the formation of carcinogens in our body. Some experts believe that chlorine may also be linked with heart disease and stroke.

Sucked in

Saccharin as a sweetener has a much longer history than the other chemicals. It has been used in foods since 1907 although somewhat sparsely at first. Shortages of sugar during World War 2 encouraged the use of this sweetener and it found a more common place within food products. Interest in saccharin rose in the early 1970's because of research that had shown that saccharin increased the rate of bladder cancer in rats. Proposals were put in place to ban the artificial sweetener, but as the only freely available no calorie sweetener at the time; this was met with strong opposition. Instead it was agreed that products containing saccharin should carry a warning label to inform the public that saccharin had been shown to cause cancer in laboratory animals. This was a compromise to allow some time for further research to be done to determine the safety of saccharin. In 1991, after 14 years, the US government formally withdrew its proposal to ban saccharin and then in 2000 removed the law requiring saccharin containing products to carry a warning label. After 23 years of saccharin being listed as a possible human carcinogen it has now been given an apparently clean bill of health. A bigger concern exists here. Despite the FDA proving the 'safety' of saccharin, they allowed a sweetener that they believed may cause cancer to continue to be ingested by the general public for 23 years! Where do their loyalties lie? In protecting public health or in protecting the financial interests of those involved in the sweetener industry?

Acesulfame K or acesulfame potassium is perhaps the least studied of the artificial sweeteners, only getting approval in 1988, and is used less than the previous three discussed. Similar to aspartame it is approximately 200 times sweeter than sugar and has a slightly bitter after taste so is often combined with other sweeteners. It is used in soft drinks, chewing gum, jellies, yoghurts, pharmaceuticals and because it is heat stable some baked goods. Some studies have shown that it causes benign tumour growths on rat thyroid glands and this of course has raised questions over its potential to be carcinogenic. It has also been shown to stimulate the release of insulin and as such increases the likelihood of causing reactive hypoglycaemia. This sweetener is often found in foods that contain low or no calories. The subsequent release of insulin will serve to push blood sugar levels down, when there was little carbohydrate pushing them upwards in the first place. This drop in blood sugar will bring on symptoms of fatigue, hunger, shakiness, clouded thinking, poor focus and loss of colour.

Nutrition's Playground

Artificial sweeteners have been used in an attempt to reduce the intake of sugar which has been shown to be detrimental to health. Whilst sugar reduction is a sensible step to take, the inclusion of artificial sweeteners in the diet increases the risk of a wide ranging number of other undesirable health effects. In the meantime the use of artificial sweeteners has continued to increase whilst sugar intake has also continued to increase. UK residents ingest 42kg of sugar per year whilst in the US nearly 65kg of sugar per year is the average. Introducing artificial sweeteners has done little to curb our sugar intake and at the same time has increased the toxic effect of manmade chemicals into our bodies.

We have been granted a sweet tooth that is greatly satisfied by eating foods with sugars in them. It is man that refined sugars in the first place and hence created the problems of excess sugar intake. Occasional intake of natural sweeteners will do little harm and still provide satisfaction to the taste buds. Here are a few suggestions that are more nutritious and less damaging

- Unheated, local honey

- Pure, organic maple syrup

- Organic coconut sugar

- Organic blackstrap molasses

- Organic rapadura (dehydrated cane sugar juice)

Not soya healthy

Soya beans have been used as a food for many years particularly in eastern parts of Asia. Claims that soya was a

Nutrition's Playground

staple food in the Asian diet and should be a mainstay as part of modern diet are not well supported despite its widespread acceptance. Soya is a major part of global food production today and has considerable commercial value. Approximately 35% of the soya bean is protein whilst 20% is oil with the remaining content being made up of carbohydrates and ash. Soya bean oil, more often referred to and sold as vegetable oil, has considerable market value and is perhaps one of the first reasons that it was grown on a vast commercial scale. The remaining husk and protein meal that was left behind from vegetable oil production served as a waste problem that was often dealt with by disposal into animal feeds. This did not make much money, but did deal with the problem. However, like all business other uses were soon discovered for the 'waste' soya meal. Today this is used to make many other food products such as soya flour; soya based infant formula, meat substitutes like textured vegetable proteins, soya milk, margarines and yoghurts. The high protein content within the bean has been commercially exploited in all of these products. Soya protein is often considered a suitable replacement for meat in those seeking to eat a more vegetable based diet.

Soya is considered by some to have a protein availability score as high as milk and eggs. There are several classifications of protein value that have been created over the years, the most common being the biological value scoring system. This is a measure out of 100 of how much protein from a food is absorbed into the body to be incorporated into cell structure and function. Biological value does have some variations that can change the score, such as the way the food is prepared and the vitamin and mineral content. Soya foods typically have a biological value between 64 and 74 compared to milk and eggs which are greater than 90. This is a result of the less digestible portions of the bean. Soya is well known as a difficult-to-digest food and this was acknowledged from the earliest references of its use in East Asian countries. For this

161

reason it was, in fact, only eaten occasionally and in some parts was even considered a poor man's food. Soya contains oligosaccharide sugars that are relatively indigestible and are responsible for the well known flatulence factor in soya foods. Soya also contains trypsin inhibitors that make protein digestion more difficult, not to mention a significant level of a compound called phytic acid. This compound has strong binding properties, the purpose of which is to protect and lock in minerals whilst the bean is waiting for optimal conditions for growth into a new plant. However they also bind valuable minerals at later stages of processing and contribute towards diminished digestibility and nutritional value.

In 1993 the World Health Organisation adopted a new protein rating system called the Protein Digestibility Corrected Amino Acid Score (PDCAAS). This new rating system compares the amino acid profile in a food to the needs of a 2-5 year old child rather than the actual levels absorbed into the body. Therefore the PDCASS does not take into account the nutritional losses excreted as a result of indigestibility, perhaps the biggest problem associated with eating soya foods. The PDCAAS rates soya protein at the highest possible rating of 1.0 the same as milk and eggs. Some feel that the wealthy soya industry helped in the formation of this new rating system in order to strengthen the case for the increasing sales of soya protein based foods and ingredients. Certainly it was one of the major food stuffs to significantly increase its rating under the new scoring system. However, the PDCAAS score does not change anything with regards to digestibility. Soya proteins are still difficult to break down and therefore have a lower value to the body compared to other protein sources such as milk and eggs.

Soya is a very potent source of isoflavones. These are plant

Nutrition's Playground

based compounds called phytoestrogens that are absorbed into the body and mimic the effects of the hormone oestrogen, the predominant female sex hormone. The body is constantly working to maintain a certain level of balance with regards to its internal chemistry. Hormones, such as oestrogen, form part of that carefully regulated balance. Oestrogen has many purposes from regulating the menstrual cycle and bone formation to managing cholesterol levels and fat deposition. Although known for stimulating female secondary sexual characteristics, oestrogen is also released in small amounts within males, though the female has many times the amount. The predominant isoflavones in soya are called genistein and daidzein. The effects of these isoflavones provide one of the common marketing angles for soya rich foods. The oestrogen mimicking effects are considered by some experts to be protective against cancer and in reducing menopausal symptoms. Other experts have raised significant concerns regarding the effects of isoflavones in disrupting hormonal balance, decreasing the function of the thyroid gland and therefore metabolism, encouraging infertility and causing some types of cancer.

Whilst soya has been a part of traditional East Asian diets for thousands of years it was only eaten in small amounts and only after particular preparation methods that made them more digestible. These low intakes had little effect on the oestrogen balance of the body compared to the much higher intakes found in modern diets where soya derived ingredients are used in many foods. Soya beans were subjected to fermentation methods over lengthy time periods in order break down indigestible components and add to its nutritional value. Traditionally fermented soy sauce, tempeh, natto and miso are examples of foods that have greater nutrient value and are less likely to disrupt the delicate balance of the body. However, they should only represent a small part of the diet rather than becoming a staple food.

Nutrition's Playground

These are a few of the more influential myths surrounding the world of nutrition, dieting and alternative health, The purpose of each of these discussions is not to highlight wrongs, but to widen understanding and provide further information that will form the basis of a more informed decision. To make a wise decision all the information must be known. Only understanding one point of view without an awareness of the other does not provide an option and therefore there is no choice. If you believe the only way to lose weight is to reduce calorie intake then that is your only course of action, either restrict your intake or remain overweight. Once a different option is provided then a choice can be made, restrict calories or improve the quality of the food being eaten. Both will lead to weight loss, but only one choice will optimise your health at the same time. The other topics discussed in this chapter will also provide you with another view and in so doing empower you with a choice. Choice is the master of change. If you want change to happen you must exercise your ability to choose with wisdom.

Nutrition's Playground

Step 7: Where There's a Will There's a Weigh

The media at large is constantly full of information regarding obesity, overweight and the national struggle to overcome it. The number of overweight and obese adults in the UK and the USA seems to be on a steady increase. Obesity rates in excess of 24% in the UK (2010) and 34% in the USA (2010) have driven weight management to the top of both governments' health agendas. However, with an even larger number falling into the overweight category almost 3 out of 4 adults over 35, it isn't just the government who have concerns. Most people who are overweight would like to lose weight and find a healthier, happier weight, yet somehow the method eludes them. It isn't for want of trying either. One of the largest surveys ever performed on dietary habits found that nearly 70% of those questioned were using diet in some way to try and manage their body weight. Between 35-40% were trying to lose weight and were using fat restriction as their method.

This suggests that many people do indeed want to lose weight and in fact a large majority are actually trying on a regular basis to do so. So why then do the rates of being overweight continue to rise despite these considerable efforts? It suggests that a successful, sure fire method has not yet been established, or those that have had some success later relapse. It may be that many of the weight loss methods used are actually the same method in disguise. The Atkins diet, Weight Watchers, the F plan, the South Beach diet, Slim Fast, the Kellogg's diet, Slimming World and the cabbage soup diet are all variations of a reduced calorie approach just promoted under a different banner.

Many ideas have been promoted as causing the major shift in weight gain in recent years, such as excess calories, processed food, fat intake, sugar intake, food additives, reduced activity, increased stress, hormonal imbalance, excess meat intake and too much carbohydrate. Which of these many 'triggers' do you remove or adjust within your diet in an attempt to lose weight? There would be little left to eat if we tried to follow them all and eating nothing is certainly a guaranteed way to lose weight! The sacrifice of health that also tends to follow severe calorie reduction would suggest it is not a sensible method. This chapter will deal with the hype and fad dieting by taking a good look at the facts found within modern science as well as those that have been known for many generations.

In the previous chapter it has already been highlighted that calorie counting is a method of weight loss that is failing those who are trying to lose weight. There are several factors that make it virtually impossible to calorie count with any accuracy. These flaws are not easily overcome outside of the scientific laboratory and so there is no choice but to consign calorie counting to the 'unsuccessful' heap. Before you revolt, claiming it made a difference to you, remember we are looking at long term success which, beyond 3 – 6 months, has been shown to be minimal in most well run scientific trials.

The first time I seriously questioned the value of calorie intake was about 4 years into my career as a health and fitness professional. I was leading a small weight loss group of 12 people on a weekly basis, guiding them through what was essentially a mainstream low fat, low calorie, increased activity approach. One particular woman on the course, let's

Nutrition's Playground

call her Joan for the sake of anonymity, was in her early fifties, about five foot tall and carrying an extra 15-20kg of weight. Joan had already been attending a mainstream diet group for several months and had been exercising at the gym 3 times a week. Frustrated at the stalemate she had reached she chose to attend our small weight loss group as well to see if there was something extra to be done. The mainstream diet group she had been attending were providing accountability via weekly support, calorie controlled targets and regular weight checks.

Initially Joan had seen success and had lost a few kilos, but this had slowed to a halt and during the previous 2 months she had become embarrassed to find each week there was no weight loss at all. Joan had continued to meet her calorie targets of only 1300 calories a day through two small meals, was attending vigorous aqua classes regularly and walking the dog on a daily basis. She knew she was doing more than others within the diet group, but was still not losing weight. At the close of our third session she came and spoke with me at the end of the meeting and described her predicament seeking some extra answer that she was not doing. I understood her frustrations, but was unsure of what more I could offer as she was doing just about everything I had been taught to do. Remembering a small article I had read about the effects of calorie restriction on slowing the metabolism I suggested that she introduce a third meal to her daily routine instead of the two small meals she was eating. After some questions I reassured her that I understood this would increase her calorie intake. Not entirely convinced this would work we came to an agreement that she would try it for 2 weeks. Joan looked me sternly in the face and warned me that if she put on any weight because of this change that she would seek me out. Knowing that I was taking a bit of a gamble with this approach I half expected Joan to show up to the gym at any point over the next two weeks ready to vent at

167

me. However, two weeks later as Joan came into our weight loss group she had a smile on her face. I had to know. Upon inquiry it turned out she had done as I asked and introduced a third meal into her daily routine which had increased her calorie intake to a little over 1600 calories. She had lost 2 – 3 pounds both weeks and was delighted. Relieved that it had worked out this began my interest in understanding how she had been able to increase her food intake and still lose weight.

The years of study and research that followed unearthed several important, though rarely understood truths regarding weight loss. These valuable considerations should be a vital part of your tactical weight loss strategy.

- Macronutrient balance
- Hormonal balancing
- Stress reduction
- Food quality

These four areas are often overlooked as part of any dietary strategy, including those adopted for the purpose of body fat reduction. Each area offers considerable benefit to overcoming excess body weight and in understanding the mechanics of how weight gain occurs in the first place.

Macronutrient balance

Macronutrients are the large energy providing nutrients in the food we eat, that is proteins, fats and carbohydrates. Various modern diets have altered the balance of these three nutrients with the claim that this makes a difference to the success of weight loss and body fat reduction. The two most common are the high carbohydrate whole food diet and the low carbohydrate Atkins style diet, which by description proves to be higher in fat. Few diets purposefully increase the

Nutrition's Playground

amount of protein above 20% of calories and this is fairly sensible as excess protein can prove to be a strain on the body. The average protein intake in the UK is between 15-16%. This may need to be increased a little for those who are very active, but for the majority, if the quality of the protein source is high, 15-20% of calories from protein will be more than adequate. Proteins have many important roles in the body including growth and repair, supporting immune responses, hormone production, enzyme and catalytic processes as well as contributing to approximately 12% of our daily energy needs.

In terms of managing weight, one of the most important roles proteins have is in stimulating as sense of satiety after a meal. All three macronutrients contribute in some way to the sense of satisfaction after eating food. Carbohydrates cause the release of certain peptide molecules from the gut that reduce hunger and bring about a feeling of satisfaction, but these naturally occurring chemicals have a relatively short lived effect. This is why many people report that if they have eaten a carbohydrate rich snack, particularly a processed snack, then 20-30 minutes later they are craving food again. The satisfaction signals that occur as a result of eating carbohydrates only have short term effects. Fats have been shown to have the least influence on satiety when eaten in isolation, but it is unlikely that many chose to eat pure oil or a lump of butter or lard on its own. Fats are usually bound up in natural foods alongside proteins. Therefore, when natural foods are eaten the limited effect of fats on feelings of satisfaction will be more than countered by the strong effects of the protein component on satiety. Proteins have been found to be the most potent stimulus for releasing gut peptides that signal to the appetite centres of the brain, to stop eating. The satiating effects of protein are much longer lasting than carbohydrates and will reduce the sense of

Nutrition's Playground

hunger and cravings considerably more than any other macronutrient.

Naturally occurring higher fat foods, as discussed, also have proteins in abundance. Meats, poultry, oily fish, eggs, dairy and nuts all contain significant amounts of both macronutrients. The high level of satiety provided by proteins in these foods will prevent overconsumption of the higher calorie fats contained within the same food product. Processed snack foods, such as biscuits, cakes, pastries, chocolate, ice cream, crisps, French fries and pizza have high levels of fats accompanied mainly by carbohydrates, not proteins. Carbohydrates have a short lived influence on satisfaction increasing the likelihood of snacking in the near future as a result of reactive low blood sugar. This is more likely to lead to what science refers to as the 'passive overconsumption' of fats in the diet. The marked increase in obesity has only happened since the increase and wide scale availability of a variety of processed, high carbohydrate, high fat snacks.

'Although dietary fat is a strong predictor of weight gain, the relationship between dietary fat and carbohydrate appears to be more relevant than fat intake alone...the combination of a fat load and a glycaemic load appears to exaggerate the insulin response and promote further weight gain.' (Isganaitis & Lustig, 2005)

The Food Standards Agency in 2006 advised the following macronutrient guidelines:

2550 calories per day for males and 1950 calories per day for females

Carbohydrates should average 50% of total calories (males 1125kcal, females 975kcal)

Nutrition's Playground

Fats no more than 35% calories (males 892kcal, females 682kcal), saturated accounting for no more than 10% (males 255kcal, females 195kcal)

Proteins make up the remaining 15% calories (males 382kcal, females 292kcal), though official guidance is 55g protein (234kcal) per day for adults

This advice has been the mainstay of what is considered a balanced diet since its inception in 1984 here in the United Kingdom. However, obesity rates in the UK have more than trebled in this same period of time rising from 7% in 1983 to 24% by 2007. This is not to say that these macronutrient ratios are the only cause, but certainly they have not of themselves provided enough control of body fat levels and obesity has risen regardless. Harvard professor Walter Willett, perhaps one of the most renowned nutrition experts in the world, published an article that caused quite a stir in 2002. In it he made a striking observation stating:

'...within the United States, a substantial decline in the percentage of energy from fat during the last 2 decades has corresponded with a massive increase in the prevalence of obesity. Diets high in fat do not appear to be the primary cause of the high prevalence of excess body fat in our society, and reductions in fat will not be a solution.'

Research published two years later by the US Centres of Disease Control and Prevention (CDC) was supportive of this statement. They found that during the period between 1971 to 2000 American obesity rates rose from 14.5% to 30.9% whilst the average calorie intake increased from 2450 – 2618 calories in males and from 1542 – 1877 calories per day in women. Carbohydrate consumption also increased in males from 42.4 - 49% of calories and in females from 45.4 - 51.6% of calories.

Nutrition's Playground

Protein consumption for the same time period was found to decrease slightly from 16.5 – 15.5% in males and from 16.9 – 15.1% in females. Surprisingly, total energy derived from fat decreased in males from 36.9 – 32.8% and from 36.1 – 32.8% in females.

When taking into account the increase in calories when calculating these new percentages, the absolute amount of fat in grams actually increased slightly 5 – 6g per day in both genders. However, this pales in comparison to the 62-68g increase in carbohydrates. The increase in fats only accounted for a 45 - 54 calorie increase, whereas the increase in carbohydrates accounted for 248 – 268 more calories. This would indicate that the increase in carbohydrates made the most significant difference in altering the energy contribution from food resulting in the doubling of obesity in the US. Despite this the total average calorie intake was not that great with males - only slightly above their recommended intake and women slightly below.

Interestingly the 2004 National Diet and Nutrition Survey in the UK found that the total levels of fat intake across the population were very similar to the guideline intake of no more than 35% calories from fat in both male and female populations. The actual percentage of calories from total fat was 35.8% for males and 34.9% for females. Carbohydrate intakes were also very close to national guidelines with males eating 47.7% and females 48.5% of calories.

A comparison of macronutrient intakes between different UK national dietary surveys collected in 1986/7 and 2000/1 published as part of National Statistics is very revealing. The table on the next page compares the different intakes between the surveys.

Nutrition's Playground

	% Total Carbohydrates	% Total Fat	% Saturated Fat	% Total protein
Males 86/87	44.7%	40.4%	16.5%	15.2%
Males 00/01	47.7%	35.8%	13.4%	16.5%
Females 86/87	44.2%	40.3%	17.0%	15.6%
Females 00/01	48.5%	34.9%	13.2%	16.6%

(Adapted from National Diet and Nutrition Survey, 2004)

This survey demonstrates some similarities to that found in the USA by the Centres of Disease Control. In both genders the percentage of carbohydrates increased whilst the percentage of fats decreased. The UK data show that the total number of calories has decreased for both genders from 2468 to 2300 in males and from 1685 to 1668 in females. Interestingly the average intake is still below the national guidelines suggesting a greater number of the population eat fewer calories than those who eat in excess. Total fat consumption has decreased approximately 200 calories in males and 180 calories in females, whilst total carbohydrate consumption has increased approximately 30 calories in males and a significant 150 calories per day in females. This means that the reduction in fat calories in women has almost been swallowed up in the increase in carbohydrate calories, hence the very small change in female total energy intake. Despite this drop in calories, decrease in fats and increase in carbohydrates, obesity levels in males rose from 8 – 21% and in females rose from 12 – 24% during the same time period that the two UK dietary surveys spanned. There is one point that is absolutely clear from this information - total fat intake cannot be directly blamed for the rise in national obesity.

Nutrition's Playground

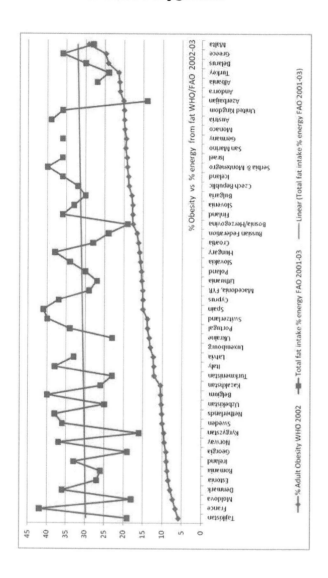

% Obesity vs % energy from fat WHO/FAO 2002-03

─── Linear (Total fat intake % energy FAO 2001-03)

─■─ Total fat intake % energy FAO 2001-03

─◆─ % Adult Obesity WHO 2002

Nutrition's Playground

Yet despite this clear data, which is freely available for the public and government to read, the prevailing dogma still encourages a low fat intake and an increase in whole carbohydrates as necessary for weight loss! Why on earth spend considerable money, time and effort to run national dietary surveys and then ignore the results they bring up?

The previous graph of European data for obesity levels and total fat intake also show a similar trend. The 51 countries are ordered from left to right in line with rising obesity rates and additionally the total amount of energy from fat is charted where data was available. The trend line only shows a difference of 2-3% of total daily calories of fat per person per day across increasing obesity rates from 6 to 29%. This represents a much weaker correlation than is normally implied in the press and public health guidelines.

Although a weak trend does exist in this data it is clear that there is huge variation in the rates of obesity compared with the total percentage of energy from fat. In fact the highest total fat intake is found in France at 42% according to this data, yet they have the second lowest obesity rate in all of Europe. This has been acknowledged by the scientific community, but is often pushed to one side as an unusual, unexplainable oddity that has become known as the French paradox. This paradox is strengthened by the fact that France also has very low rates of heart disease to match. However, it is not the only 'paradox' present in Europe. Belgium, Switzerland and Spain also eat 40% or more of their calories as fat and are found in the lower half of European obesity rates.

The paradox seems to work the other way around in some cases too. Azerbaijan has the lowest total fat intake out of all 51 European nations, but has the 7th highest obesity rate. Bosnia Herzegovina, Turkey and the Russian Federation all

Nutrition's Playground

eat less than 25% total calories from fat and are found in the top half of European obesity rates. It must be accepted that evidence exists that does not agree with the theory that high dietary fat intakes cause overweight and obesity.

It is very difficult to locate suitable information on carbohydrate ingestion and obesity levels as this is rarely collated as a complete statistic in the majority of dietary surveys. Usually information collected is related to carbohydrate food sources such as fruit and vegetables, sugars, grains and potatoes rather than the actual amount of carbohydrate. WHO and FAO data on these foods is available. Sugar, grain and potato consumption figures surprisingly show no correlation with rising rates of obesity. However, somewhat controversially, the FAO data on fruit and vegetable consumption in grams per person per day shows a strong positive correlation with rising obesity. The following graph shows the comparison between fruit and vegetable intake and obesity. As in the previous graph the 51 countries are ordered with obesity increasing from left to right.

Fruit and vegetables clearly contribute to total calorie intake just as fats do which may go some way to explaining this unexpected pattern. The main macronutrient present in most fruit and vegetables is carbohydrate, though it must be acknowledged that the majority of fruit and vegetables tend not to be particularly dense in calories compared to other foods. The trend line does cover a spread of nearly 200 grams per person per day, a significant 800 calorie energy difference. Similarly to the previous graph there are some countries that don't fall in line with this unexpected trend. Belarus and the Czech Republic have high obesity rates and low fruit and vegetable consumption, whilst the opposite is observed in France, Italy and Portugal.

Nutrition's Playground

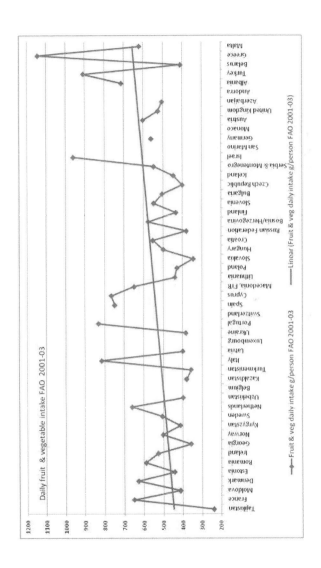

Nutrition's Playground

This investigation into population wide obesity and macronutrient contributions shows that obesity can occur in many different ways. There are always several exceptions to the rule at both ends of the spectrum. Therefore, it must be accepted that there is no guarantee with regards to certain dietary patterns and the appearance of obesity. The following comparison of the United Kingdom and Azerbaijan highlights two countries with significant differences in dietary intake, but yet virtually identical obesity rates. These two nations had obesity rates in 2001 averaging 20% in the UK and 20.15% in Azerbaijan. The shaded box indicates which country has the highest intake in each category.

The only similar figures found across all categories compared above are fruit and vegetable intake. Total calories, fat intake, sugar, potatoes and protein intake are all different with the UK consuming more in every case. Azerbaijan does have about a 57% higher prevalence of diabetes than the UK and a much higher cereal intake. Could this large cereal intake be the reason Azerbaijan has a virtually identical level of obesity to the UK even though they eat fewer calories and total fat? It is unlikely we will ever know the reason for such different intakes, yet similar obesity outcomes. The point to accept here is that we cannot assume that obesity is caused just through excess calories or too much fat in the diet.

	Obese (%)	Fruit & veg (g)	Fat (g)	Kcal	Sugar (g)	Grain (g)	Potato (g)	Protein (g)
U K	20	526	138	3449	112.3	312.3	347.9	103
Azb	20.15	506	41	2643	46.6	583.6	178.1	77

Nutrition's Playground

Understanding the cause of obesity may actually be different to understanding the solution. The human body is a complex organism controlled by multiple regulating systems. Excess calories from dietary fat, protein, fruit, vegetables and alcohol are likely to be a part of the equation to becoming overweight or obese. However, that does not mean that a simple reduction in any one of these components will reverse the situation. Consider the following analogy. If a tap is left running the bath will soon overflow and start to flood the room. Simply turning off the tap prevents the situation getting worse, but does not reduce the volume of water inside the bath. You would be foolish to jump in at this point as the water will flood out. A different action altogether is required. The plug needs to be pulled out for a time until a satisfactory water level is reached, only then can you climb in and relax. A completely different action to the root cause may be required to resolve excess weight problems. Understanding the triggers is helpful in obesity prevention, but other considerations need to be taken into account when obesity has already occurred and a solution is sought.

'...dietary fat may be particularly important in inducing obesity, whereas a reduction in dietary fat has less of an effect on weight loss.' (Bray & Popkin, 1998)

The evidence supporting dietary fat as the main cause of overweight and obesity is certainly not conclusive and according to some evidence is quite weak. In fact population wide surveys and historical observations of indigenous population groups who ate large amounts of fat do not illustrate the theory that fat causes obesity. The Masai, Eskimo and Native Americans ate very high fat diets yet did not exhibit high levels of obesity. The Masai and Native Americans were particularly known for being lean and strong on their high animal fat diets. It is also worth considering that the dominant fat sources in the modern diet have changed considerably as well during the course of the last 40 - 50 years with a clear move away from animal based fats and a considerable increase in the use of seed and bean oils, much of which is solidified by a process called hydrogenation. Therefore, it may not even be appropriate to compare total fat intake across populations as the types being eaten have changed so much over the years. This is quite a complex topic with many varied arguments. Having reviewed the wide and varied evidence regarding dietary fat and obesity Bray and Popkin concluded:

'There is some evidence that a low fat diet may be protective to specific sub groups of the population, and hence, be more relevant to obesity in a preventative than a treatment perspective...it must be kept in mind that low fat diets offer no panacea, since individuals with a predisposition to over eating appear to learn how to do so, even on fat reduced diets.'

Hormonal balancing

Despite commonly held beliefs that obesity is caused primarily by excessive eating and sedentary behaviours it has become well accepted that certain hormones play a significant part in the cause of obesity and without their controlling influence obesity and overweight would be less likely to occur.

The Insulin key

The human body has many hormones to control the internal environment. There are numerous hormones involved in fat breakdown, but only a few with any influence on fat storage. Insulin is considered the primary hormone in the human body that governs the storage of body fat, yet it is rarely

Nutrition's Playground

discussed in this context. It is normally only mentioned in understanding the control of blood sugar.

Insulin is secreted by a small organ that sits just below the stomach called the pancreas. Insulin is released in response to the presence of carbohydrates, and to a lesser extent proteins, in a meal. Fats cause little response from the pancreas with almost no insulin output. When blood sugar levels rise insulin is released into circulation and interacts on both muscle and fat cells. The activated cells open small channels allowing for the movement of glucose into the interior of the cells. This facilitates the use of glucose within the cells for immediate energy, for storage as complex carbohydrate or for conversion to fats both for energy or storage. Each of these processes is considered a normal and healthy response to a meal.

To more fully understand the role of insulin in fat storage we need to understand how the fat cell functions. The primary function of the fat cell is the storage or release of energy. The notion that fat is trapped within fat tissue is incorrect as this tissue is always in a state of flux. The main consideration is which direction the net movement is taking place.

'Over a 2-3 week period, all of the stored triglycerides (fats) in an adipose cell (fat cell) have been turned over, that is catabolised for energy production or broken down into free fatty acids to be reformed into new triglyceride molecules.' (Lack, 2009)

To try and understand the way that we store and release fats we need to get a little bit technical. Fats travel in the blood stream in a form known as a triglyceride. Fats are also stored in the fat cells as triglycerides. However, they cannot pass into or out of the fat cell as a triglyceride. Triglyceride molecules are too large and need to be broken down into their smaller component parts, fatty acids and glycerol, in order to pass through the channels in the fat cell membrane. Only the smaller fatty acids are able to pass through the narrow channels into the fat cell. In order to be rebuilt into a triglyceride the fatty acids must be re-connected to the carbohydrate backbone, glycerol that was left behind on the other side of the cell membrane. As glycerol does not enter the fat cell the body needs to draw on another source. This molecular backbone can only be created inside the fat cell when sufficient glucose is allowed to enter the fat cell and is converted into the needed glycerol component. This enables the rebuilding of the triglyceride within the fat cell for storage. Fats can only be stored in their triglyceride form and as such can only be stored when sufficient glucose is available to the cells. Therefore, both carbohydrates and the related response from insulin are essential for the formation of and storage of triglycerides within the fat cell. It is vital that this is understood. If we eat large amounts of fat in the diet there will certainly be greater movement of fatty acids into both fat and muscle cells. However, as long as they remain in their fatty acid form they cannot be locked into the fat cell and as a result will be able to move freely in and out of the cell when needed. Fats must be converted into a triglyceride for longer term storage and this can only happen when there are carbohydrates present to allow a glucose supply into the fat cell for glycerol formation.

Excess blood glucose and high levels of triglyceride circulating in the blood promote a condition known as insulin resistance. When cellular needs for glucose have been met or the body has released an abundance of fatty acids into circulation there is no longer any need for the passage of glucose into the cells. This leads to the closing of channels particularly on muscle cell membranes until such a time as the need for glucose increases again. The more often these blood parameters are pushed upwards beyond cellular requirements the greater the signal to close the channels becomes. Over years this can lead to a build up of resistance to the hormonal signal insulin provides to open the cellular channels. This means that despite an intake of carbohydrates in a meal and a normal rise in blood insulin the cells do not respond as usual and glucose remains in the blood rather than being allowed to pass into muscle tissue. Interestingly the fat cells still retain their sensitivity for insulin far beyond the time that the muscles become resistant. This means that glucose can still pass into fat cells to be utilised and stored whilst at the same time muscle cells are only allowing minimal uptake.

'Adipose (fat) tissue tends to retain its sensitivity to insulin in the face of ... skeletal muscle resistance.' (Isganaitis & Lustig, 2005)

This muscular resistance to insulin leads to the pancreas having no choice but to respond continually to the elevated blood glucose by increasing its production of insulin following ingestion of carbohydrates to even higher levels in an attempt to open cellular channels. Muscle tissue is normally responsible for accepting the majority of ingested glucose, perhaps as much as 70%. In the insulin resistant state muscle cells are inhibited from accepting as much, which leaves fat cells to manage a larger amount of incoming glucose. This increases the amount of fat stored as triglyceride within the fat cells by shifting the net flux of fatty acid movement, whilst at the same time inhibiting the release of fatty acids from the fat cells.

'Experimental and clinical studies are gradually painting a picture in which obesity promotes insulin resistance, and insulin resistance conversely facilitates further weight gain.' (Isganaitis & Lustig, 2005)

Nutrition's Playground

It has been suggested that the association with obesity and insulin resistant muscle tissue occurs simultaneously with another apparent association, obesity and insulin resistance in the brain. Insulin release has been shown to lower the addictive potential of a pleasurable stimulus or food. Therefore, under normal conditions the release of insulin quickly satisfies and reduces the need or craving for a food. It decreases the foods addictive drive by blunting the receptors in the brain. This is because food has just been ingested to provide the insulin release and the body is switching off its appetite mechanisms in response. The brain conveniently uses insulin to serve as an 'off' switch. An overweight or obese individual who demonstrates insulin resistance to muscle tissue is also likely to experience insulin resistance to the brain. This will prevent insulin from reaching the areas of the brain normally affected and it will not be able to inhibit this drive for palatable foods. Insulin, the 'off' switch, is unable to reach its needed destination and appetite remains elevated longer than in a non-insulin resistant individual. This sets the stage for an unchecked drive to eat even in the face of excess calorie intake. Insulin resistance is becoming a considerable part of the obesity problem. This is evident by the increasing rates of abdominal or apple shaped obesity that has been observed in recent years. Insulin resistance has been strongly correlated with increased storage of fat around the abdomen and the internal organs. The fat cells in this region are able to 'process' greater amounts of fatty acids and glucose than fat cells in other regions of the body if the environment is right. Insulin resistance creates the right environment and hence leads to abdominal obesity.

It stands to reason that reducing abdominal obesity must include the necessary steps to control chronically elevated levels of insulin in the blood stream. As the most potent stimulus of insulin, carbohydrates must be reduced in those who are overweight. National dietary surveys show that in

Nutrition's Playground

the majority of the population carbohydrate intake accounts for approximately 50% of our daily calories. Combined with the encouragement to eat little and often this has lead to regular bursts in blood glucose and therefore blood insulin, which continues to perpetuate the fat storing internal environment found in those with insulin resistance. Reducing the number of calories from carbohydrates, particularly starchy carbohydrates such as bread, pasta, rice, grains and potatoes, to between 20-40% of total daily intake will serve to reduce blood glucose levels and in time reverse the process of insulin resistance.

Daily carbohydrates should be ingested in the form of fresh, seasonal vegetables, non-starchy beans and legumes and occasional fruit when it is in season. This will provide vital nutrients to optimise health, but without such a powerful stimulus for insulin production. This may initially be a difficult step to take for those who have become dependent on carbohydrates for the bulk of their daily calories. Ingrained habits and behaviours can be difficult to break. Successfully making these changes will be discussed in later chapters

Oestrogen and testosterone

Oestrogen and testosterone production increase naturally in males and females as a consequence of reaching puberty and the physical changes leading to adulthood. During these years males generally increase their bone density and lean muscle tissue and experience a reduction in body fat mass whilst testosterone levels are increasing. Females increase in bone and muscle tissue, but also increase the storage of body fat at particular sites, the main regions being the hips, buttocks, thighs and around the breasts. These physical changes, including the increase in body fat around the hips and thighs, are driven by rising oestrogen during this period. The same pattern can also be observed during pregnancy when oestrogen levels increase to stimulate and support the growth of the uterus and foetus, but also serve to increase body fat deposits around the hips and thighs even more. This fat deposit acts as an energy reservoir that the mother draws upon during lactation to feed the new baby. It has also been observed that this specific body fat store often decreases during the weeks and months of lactation as the energy reserve is depleted. The change that sex hormones cause in body fat levels occurs during puberty regardless of fluctuations in energy intake.

Once past puberty and into adulthood both testosterone and oestrogen, when maintained within healthy balance, stimulate fat burning and help to prevent excess fat accumulation. Obesity and overweight can result when these sex steroids slip out of balance as part of a chain of hormonal events. In circumstances where levels of circulating oestrogen in a female's body are elevated over a longer period of time it can bring about negative effects with regards to body fat tissue. Elevated oestrogen has been found to decrease fat mass stored around the internal organs, which is beneficial in lowering the risk of chronic health conditions like heart disease and diabetes. However, regarding weight gain it has been found in adult females to cause a specific regional increase in fat storage around the hips, buttocks and thighs. This over time can lead to an increase in the typical 'pear-shaped' body more dominant in females, referred to as a gynoid pattern of overweight or obesity. Fat tissue in this region has been shown to have a greater density of cellular receptors that respond to oestrogen in the blood stream. This may go some way to explaining why this female dominant pattern exists.

Nutrition's Playground

There are several modern factors which may perturb the oestrogenic balance in females, elevating levels beyond normal and increasing the fat deposits in a typical pear-shaped pattern. These factors include:

- Pharmaceutical contraceptives

- Xenoestrogens

- Phytoestrogens

The combined contraceptive pill releases a blend of oestrogen and progestin for each of the 21 days of the 28 day menstrual cycle that they are taken. This is an effective way of preventing pregnancy by creating the wrong internal environment for a fertilised egg to embed in the lining of the uterus, the egg eventually being flushed out. In order to achieve this, the contraceptive pill elevates oestrogen beyond normal levels. Hormones are non-specific chemicals that always have multiple areas of influence when they are released into the blood stream. The oestrogen boosting contraceptive pill will not only affect the uterus and ovaries, but will also stimulate the fat cell receptors around the body. This may potentially lead to increase in fat storage around the hips, thighs and buttocks in females where there is a greater density of oestrogen cellular receptors. Interestingly weight gain is a listed side effect of taking the contraceptive pill. This may also be a side effect of excess oestrogen that has been elevated through other stimuli.

Xenoestrogens are industrially made compounds that have an oestrogen mimicking effect in the human body. They have similar effects in the body as natural oestrogens and so assist in bringing about growth of the endometrium and breast tissue. They have been implicated in some studies as increasing the likelihood of both endometrial and breast cancer. Chemicals that have been shown to contain xenoestrogens are wide and varied, but include parabens, phthalates, polychlorinated biphenyls (PCB's), bisphenol A and many pesticides. Parabens are found in many lotions, makeup and hair products. Phthalates and bisphenol A are found in many plastics, which leech out more easily the softer the plastic is or the warmer it becomes. PCB's are found in lubricants, adhesives and paints. Whilst pesticides are used freely on industrially grown crops that do not follow organic principles. Therefore, women who regularly use make up and beauty products, warm and cook food in plastic containers in the microwave, who have recently redecorated their home and eat non-organic industrial food will be exposed to many sources of xenoestrogens that will surely have an influence. Xenoestrogens may also influence the storage of fat within gynoid regions, the same as naturally occurring oestrogen does, and as such may need to be minimised in those with a pear shaped appearance. Changing to only natural beauty products and toiletries, avoiding plastic wrapped food and warming food in plastic containers and even purchasing organic foods that don't allow routine pesticide use will go a considerable way to minimising the toxic effects of xenoestrogens.

Phytoestrogens are a group of naturally occurring non-steroidal plant compounds that are similar in structure to active oestrogen, and as such have the ability to exhibit oestrogenic effects. The most researched are a compound called isoflavones which are found in very high amounts in soy products and also in smaller amounts in many foods such as linseed, sesame seed, oats, lentils and other dried beans. Research around phytoestrogens is complex with many scientists claiming they are beneficial to health, whilst other studies suggesting health concerns. There is no doubt that they can elevate oestrogen in the body. However, whether

Nutrition's Playground

there is a benefit to health may have more to do with an individual's current oestrogen balance.

A woman lacking in oestrogen may find some benefit which may be why many women passing through menopause find improvements in the symptoms experienced at this time in life when they eat foods with isoflavones or take a suitable supplement. This gives rise to the question of why you would want to elevate oestrogen levels when menopause is the natural time the female body tries to decrease oestrogen as part of ending the reproductive period. Women of reproductive age who have been regularly exposed to sources of oestrogen as explained earlier would unlikely benefit from eating foods that will serve to boost already elevated oestrogen. Yet unscrupulous companies, looking to increase profit margins, market isoflavones in foods or in supplements as being vital for female health. These circumstances may warrant the avoidance of the most potent source of phytoestrogens, soy products, when guiding female clients with existing pear shaped weight problems.

The more prevailing problem regarding obesity and health centres on the levels of testosterone in both males and females and the imbalances that may exist. Testosterone in conjunction with growth hormone stimulates fat burning in a very effective, 'powerful and multifaceted manner' (Bjorntorp, 1997). Evidence suggests that in males obesity is associated with diminished levels of testosterone. Testosterone receptor density is much higher in fat tissue surrounding the internal organs and so the most common obesity pattern observed in males with low testosterone is one of abdominal obesity. As testosterone levels drop, this results in reduced protection against fat deposits around the belly, allowing for fat accumulation in preference to fat burning.

Nutrition's Playground

Females can also develop and store body fat more centrally. This can happen at any stage of life, but tends to be more common during menopause and in the years leading up to this stage of life. Prior to menopause oestrogen tends to be the dominant hormone, as we have discussed, offering some protection against increasing central weight gain. Menopause brings about the reduction of oestrogen as the body naturally prepares to cease the menstrual cycle and the fertile reproductive period of life. The reduction in oestrogen also leads to a parallel reduction in the protection against body fat gain around the internal organs. With oestrogen from the ovaries diminishing the levels of testosterone in the female body now become relatively higher as the adrenal glands continue to produce this hormone. Elevated testosterone in the female does the exact opposite of what it does in males, and together with increased insulin resistance brings about central weight gain. This increase in central body fat in females can also occur prior to menopause and would typically still be associated with elevated insulin and higher testosterone to oestrogen balance. Central fat accumulation brings about the same disease risk characteristics in females as would be expected in the male overweight population. Reducing starchy carbohydrates would also be beneficial for women passing through menopause as this would reduce glucose in the blood and decrease the chances of more permanently adding to abdominal weight gain.

Stressed out and out of cortisol

Cortisol is the major hormone released from the adrenal glands primarily in response to stress. Cortisol has many effects, the majority of which serve to support and protect the body during times of stress. Above all it serves to increase energy by releasing stored sugar and fatty acids into the blood stream. This purpose has lead to cortisol being referred to as a catabolic hormone as structures are being broken down to release energy. This makes cortisol a powerful fat burning hormone. Modern living has greatly influenced the amount of stress we are subjected to on a daily basis. Almost from the moment we wake up until we go to sleep at night there is a constant barrage of stress inducing events that call upon the adrenal glands to release cortisol and its sister hormone, adrenaline. Consider the following possible events in the life of an individual who commutes to the city:

Early morning alarm clock – sudden awakening

Quick breakfast of coffee and toast – caffeine and blood sugar hit

Rush to the train station and the cramped journey to work

Work in a middle management position – staff to oversee below and senior staff to please above

10.30am dip in performance – fatigue leads to more coffee

Too busy to stop for lunch – work through with cheap

sandwich, crisps and soft drink

2pm dip in performance, feel fatigued – more coffee

4pm dip in performance, feel fatigued – more coffee

Work late to meet deadlines, hungry by this time – leave at 6.30pm

Hectic journey home on cramped train

Nutrition's Playground

Desperate to eat, really hungry – quick snack the moment arrive home – biscuits & beer/wine

Prepare microwave ready meal – eat in front of the television

Watch an action movie to unwind with some more beer/wine

Fall into bed late and wake up between 1am-3am to go to bathroom – poor sleeping patterns

Every one of the events listed above induces an element of stress on the human body and as such will stimulate the release of cortisol from the adrenal glands. How long can such a lifestyle be maintained? Yet for many this is the type of lifestyle they lead. Some, if not all, of these bulleted points form a regular daily part of modern life. The body can respond to these stresses through the adrenal response very well, but the longer this type of unrelenting pattern continues the more the body drains its resources and the more difficult it is for the adrenals to keep up, especially with the poor nutrition provided from modern foods. Over time when the adrenals start to struggle to maintain the regular stimulus that is required of them, a condition called adrenal fatigue may result. The brain continues to release hormones to stimulate adrenal function in direct relation to the stress experienced, but the adrenals, worn down over time, struggle to meet the demand to release the required amount of cortisol. The adrenals are basically burned out!

'10% of the population...display a 'burn-out' condition...cortisol secretion is about 75% of controls...cortisol secretion in this condition is associated with central obesity and its well known associated risk factors.' (Bjorntorp, 2001)

Nutrition's Playground

Whilst this lack lustre adrenal function only occurs in one out of every 10 people there are many who are unknowingly working hard at driving their adrenals into the ground and it is likely that these figures will continue to rise as we carry on living a non-stop modern lifestyle. Adrenal fatigue usually follows a period of chronic cortisol excess and elevated daily stress patterns. Numerous studies have investigated daily cortisol release patterns across the population. Older population groups experience higher daily cortisol concentrations. These differences are strongest, and considered statistically significant, throughout the afternoon and during the early hours of the morning whilst they are asleep. Elevated cortisol levels are also higher in those with heavier body weights compared to leaner individuals. Most studies also report higher levels of cortisol found in men compared to women which falls in line with greater central weight gain in men than women. This indicates that the most likely group to experience elevated cortisol are older males. Females in many cases experience elevated cortisol and abdominal weight gain though this is more likely after menopause when oestrogen drops and testosterone levels are relatively higher.

The antidote to cortisol burn out is to introduce restorative and relaxing periods into your daily cycle in conjunction with quality nutrition and improved sleep patterns. The extent of the stressful rollercoaster today is usually met with worn out people who look to respond with costly steps to get some relaxation, a holiday abroad, a full pamper day at a spa, regular massage treatments, drinking with friends at the local bar and other such similar actions. The expense incurred at some point induces more stress to earn the money necessary to pay for such activities. Alcohol may on face value appear to provide a relaxing and stress relieving effect on a person, but the reality is the kidneys and liver have to increase their workload significantly in order to detoxify the system.

193

Nutrition's Playground

Alcohol intake has also been shown to increase the intake of food by approximately 12% and the choices of food when under the influence are consistently of lower quality. Poor quality foods also add to the stress placed on the body. Alcohol may send you into a stupor of sleep, but once again it negatively affects sleep patterns and doesn't allow the individual to get into their restorative deep sleep phases during the night. This further stresses the body and keeps cortisol elevated at night when it should be at its lowest.

In order to manage stress appropriately actions that support adrenal function and provide restorative time for the body will serve dividends. Cortisol is made originally from cholesterol which undergoes a number of conversions during its formation. Whilst much of our cholesterol is made by the liver the body needs vitamin A in abundance in order to manage each chemical conversion and reach the end product, the cortisol that is released from the adrenal glands. Vitamin A is a fat soluble nutrient suggesting that a high quality diet with appropriate fats should be eaten to support cholesterol requirements and provide vitamin A in appropriate supply. Vitamin A always needs to be taken in a suitable ratio with vitamin D in order to ensure good function, a balance which many scientists now suggest should be 5 units of vitamin A for every 1 unit of vitamin D. The daily average requirement of vitamin A is 5000 IU making the harmonising need for vitamin D 1000 IU. This can be difficult to get right through diet alone and may be easier to take in supplement form. The best quality cod liver oil is balanced in this ratio of A to D.

One of cortisol's major functions is to maintain blood sugar levels by releasing energy stored in the body. When the adrenal glands are not performing adequately this can influence these normally, tightly controlled parameters. It is also common in those who experience a lot of stress in their lives that they push themselves to accomplish more and as a result may not eat for long periods of time because they are so focused on their work or other objectives. These long spells without food only serve to lower blood sugar even more increasing internal stressors, which in turn create a greater need for cortisol release to raise flagging blood sugar. In those with adrenal fatigue cortisol cannot be produced at the level needed and so individuals may experience intense cravings for sweet food as a learned reaction to low blood sugar. Regular sugary snacks will certainly increase blood sugar, but often too quickly and too much. This of course pushes blood insulin too high and shifts the body towards fat storage. This eating pattern creates a difficult cycle to break. Low blood sugar, hunger and fatigue lead to intense cravings and reactive eating of sugary foods which rapidly raise insulin levels and shift the body into a fat storing state. Increasing body fat leads to insulin resistance which in turn reduces the glucose available to the muscle tissue and therefore reduces cellular energy production leading to even more hunger and fatigue. This behavioural pattern can be very difficult to break, especially when it has not been identified and an appropriate plan instigated to bring about positive change.

Time for stress

Timing meals is very important in those experiencing burned out adrenals. It is fairly common behaviour in those with this condition to go long periods between eating and falling into a vicious cycle of cravings and fat storage. Despite low appetite early in the morning it is essential that a quality breakfast is eaten before 10am in the morning to provide balance and nutrients for the working day. The earliest point at which appetite perks up and food can be eaten should be allocated for breakfast no matter how small it may be, just as long as it is of good quality. This should be followed up with an early lunch rather than pushing the limits of 'between meal' endurance, usually prior to 12 noon is best. A mid afternoon snack between 2-3pm will usually help sustain you through the dip in cortisol that normally occurs between 3-4pm when many feel tired and fatigued. Where possible your main meal should be eaten before 6pm which, for most who battle with stress, will bring about a lift in the evening which is often where the 'stressed out' actually feel their best, most balanced and energetic. Finally a good quality snack prior to sleeping is often helpful in stabilising blood sugar during the night and helping lower cortisol levels that will assist in improving the quality of sleep.

A reduction in starchy and sugary carbohydrates is often needed for those who are prone to stress even though those with adrenal fatigue often suffer with low blood sugar. Those with burned out adrenals once had plenty of energy and in an effort to find fuel to tap into again it is common to turn to foods that energise at the expense of the adrenals such as coffee, cola, sweet snacks and fast food. The body soon picks up that high fat foods provide more sustained energy and the individual seeks out high fat and refined carbohydrate fast foods. The problem here is the food is of poor quality in all departments and does little to provide any nutrition to rebuild adrenal health. It is the wrong grade of fuel to put in the tank and as a result leads to sluggish performance. It is much better to ensure there is an adequate amount of quality protein, fats and some carbohydrates at every meal and every snack. The benefit here is that each of these food groups is digested and fed into your blood stream at different rates maintaining better overall levels of blood glucose and therefore more sustained energy.

Carbohydrates are absorbed quickest, but as they have been cut back to smaller amounts they don't lift blood sugar too high to push insulin up and lead to further fat storage. Proteins take longer and fats sustain the longest. This seems like very simple advice but takes some thought to put into practice. Consider a typical breakfast that includes foods like breakfast cereal with skimmed milk, toast, sweetened low fat yoghurt, fruit or fruit juice. We have been conditioned to eat these foods through national food guidelines and television advertising at this particular time of day. All these foods are carbohydrate dominant, they will briefly energise, but by mid morning blood sugar levels will be flagging and cravings and appetite will strongly direct future food choices towards sweets, crisps, soft drinks and coffee to get the needed boost. Most snacks during the day tend to be carbohydrate dominant too with foods like fruit, cereal bars, cakes, biscuits, crisps and soft drinks. Those experiencing low adrenal function tend to be made worse with fruit intake mainly due to the fructose content and high potassium found in many fruits.

Protein intake should constitute a part of every meal. It is fairly common for those who have adrenal fatigue to suffer with low levels of hydrochloric acid production in their stomach. This can make one feel bloated, heavy and experience gas after a meal with protein. This often leads people to reduce the protein in their food and rely more on carbohydrates as they do not experience the same post meal effects. This only serves to compound the problem by straining the adrenals with higher blood sugar and the subsequent crash. Quality protein is a vital part of supporting the adrenals. Therefore, it is a much more effective strategy to help the body produce more hydrochloric acid prior to a meal containing protein to aid digestion, than to avoid proteins and compound the problem with high carbohydrate foods forming the bulk of the meal. A simple solution can be to dilute 2 tablespoons of cider vinegar in some water and drink 10 minutes prior to a meal to help in the production and support of stomach acids. This will help in protein digestion. If this seems to have little effect then the next option will be to take some supplemental hydrochloric acid tablets to increase the acid levels in the gut. These should be taken carefully as too many can create a warmth and burning sensation. If this is experienced then you must reduce your intake to a level where this warmth does not happen.

Routine eating habits can be difficult to change as they require a break in the cycle followed by the introduction of more sustainable alternatives that will provide benefit to the body rather than continuing the onslaught on the adrenals. Breakfast that constitutes porridge made from pre-soaked oats, whole milk, butter and a little quality salt eaten after a single boiled egg will do a much better job of sustaining blood sugar through to lunch time than any manufactured breakfast cereal. An apple with a good size chunk of cheese or a handful of nuts and dried fruit is a much more satisfying snack that will last beyond the next 30 minutes.

Another routine habit worth breaking is to stop being afraid of salt. In an earlier chapter it was highlighted how most salt is processed to the point that little goodness is left in the product. That is not the salt the body needs. It is the unprocessed, hand-harvested, grey sea salt that will be of huge benefit in nourishing tired adrenals. Often those with adrenal fatigue will have low blood pressure and quality salt will help normalise this. Low cortisol levels affect another hormone called aldosterone which helps to regulate sodium balance and other minerals. When aldosterone levels drop the body draws sodium out of the cells into the blood and excretes this through urination. This leads to low cellular and blood sodium levels which must be restored, hence the common craving for salty foods in those with burned out adrenals.

Ensuring that good quality food is eaten is such a vital component in nourishing the human body and therefore

Nutrition's Playground

managing excess weight that the whole of the next chapter is devoted to understanding this topic. Managing excess body weight can be difficult and as there is no guaranteed formula it can take some trial and error to find what works best. The diet industry makes vast sums of money each year trying to provide the answer to weight loss for those stuck in their own overweight bodies. Yet for so many serial dieters these off the shelf diet packages rarely provide the long term answer. Initial weight loss that is so often identified as 'success' in the majority of cases results in regaining that weight 3-6 months down the line when the body has adjusted to the caloric restriction that was imposed. Maybe we should stop calling it weight loss, because when we lose something we usually try to find it again as seems to be the case with excess body weight.

Stepping off the calorie counting rollercoaster, altering the balance of macronutrients, understanding and manipulating the current hormonal balance, managing stress in all its forms and optimising food quality will provide a much more stable foundation for the body to shift towards health and release the excess stored body fat. After all, if the body is healthy it won't be threatened and store extra energy for survival. Being overweight is a sign of less than optimal health rather than only an inconvenient mass that affects how we look. So many people achieve some degree of weight loss, but sacrifice health and well being in the process. If you look slim but are tired, moody and get easily stressed then health is clearly still beyond your grasp. This is a recipe for failure in the long term.

A shift in attitude away from weight loss to focus on bringing the body into a state of optimal health will have greater benefit and lead to long term weight management as a desirable side effect of the great health that is achieved. A healthy body won't be too tired, nor experience periods of

Nutrition's Playground

hyperactivity. A healthy body won't leave you depressed in the morning and feeling elated in the evening. A healthy body won't leave you lacking energy throughout the day, then wide awake in bed desperate to sleep at night. A healthy female body won't suffer terrible pre-menstrual syndrome nor store excess body fat around the hips and thighs. A healthy male body won't lose its temper on the flip of a coin or store all its body fat directly on the belly. A healthy body will be alert in the morning with a positive outlook for the new day. A healthy body will consistently have energy available to meet life's demands. A healthy body will have balanced emotions that can be managed and controlled. A healthy body will have a routine appetite and rarely have cravings. A healthy body will experience an enjoyable, refreshing daily sleep cycle. Ultimately a healthy body will easily maintain an optimal weight that is neither too thin nor too fat.

Excess weight has one major characteristic - it loves to be the centre of attention. When you get dressed in the morning, when you are out with friends, when you are shopping for clothes, when you eat a meal, when you try to exercise and when you are home at night, being overweight always ensures its presence is known. Excess weight, just like a spoilt, naughty child, relentlessly occupies your time, thoughts and your emotions if you continue to give it the attention it so craves. Optimal health is like a well behaved, quiet child that unintentionally gets forgotten about because the naughty child occupies all the available attention. So, can we agree on this? Stop trying to lose weight and begin seeking out optimal health and you will be surprised how quickly excess weight slips away and stops bothering you when it is no longer the focus of your attention. Spend some time focusing on optimal health it is much more enjoyable and rewarding. Decide today to make a difference.

Nutrition's Playground

Step 8: Quality Counts

Over the years I have seen many television programmes, read many nutrition articles in magazines and attended many health, fitness and nutrition conventions and rarely has the subject of food quality been properly discussed. The common view taken regarding food quality is to stop eating processed, convenience and fast foods and to eat more grains, fruit and vegetables. I am not denying that this is a sensible change, but this approach has not really talked about food quality, rather it has altered the foods being eaten which, by default, may have improved the quality of the food.

Food quality is probably one of the most important aspects of turning our focus towards optimal health. Once you become passionate about this subject and seek out the best foods you can afford it is amazing how many people really begin to enjoy their food again. Food stops being something you loathe because it causes you to become overweight, it stops being something that simply fuels you through the day and it stops being your emotional companion to help you through times when you are depressed or frustrated. Focusing on food quality becomes a discovery of beautiful tastes, aromas, delicious recipes, enjoyable meals and rather than food preparation being a chore, it becomes a truly pleasurable experience. In order to fully understand what brings quality and nutrition to food we first need to understand the cyclic nature of food production, where it begins and the stages along the way that either adds to the nutritional value or takes away from it.

Nutrition's Playground

As we are the top of the food chain in the vast majority of cases, the cycle of food quality begins in the soil and ends when man eats the food. The steps of the cycle are as follows:

- The quality of nutrients and micro-organisms in the soil determine

- the quality of the plants that grow in the soil, which determine

- the quality of the animals that eat the plants, which determine

- the quality of food harvested or slaughtered by man, which provides

- the starting point of nutrient degradation through industrial food handling, which determines

- the quality of food eaten by man, which determines

- the health and vitality of man, who ultimately decides

- how to enrich the soil and rear the animals that serve as our food.

It is clear from this cycle that mankind can greatly benefit from a well managed food cycle that nurtures and protects the valuable nutrients naturally formed through honouring the stages of progression. How we manage the soil, grow our plants and rear our animals determines the peak nutrient content of our food. If these early steps are managed poorly the peak nutrient density of food will be low and it will matter little how 'natural' or unprocessed our food is as the

Nutrition's Playground

levels of nutrients will not be sufficient. When the soils are lacking in nutrients and micro-organisms they begin to lose the valuable topsoil that many plant species rely on to nourish them. This topsoil is also a perfect medium for retaining water, so when it is lacking the soil becomes dry and parched. Dry, nutrient depleted soils cannot grow plants of any decent quality. In the cycle it is man who determines how to enrich the soil and we have quickly understood that this poor soil cannot sustain plant life very well. To remedy this problem man has created fertilisers and advanced irrigation systems.

Fertilisers provide the basic minerals needed by plants to sustain growth, but tend to make the soil too acidic or alkaline for micro-organisms to flourish. This does not solve the problem of depleted soils and so only provides a temporary solution to depleted soils. Plants grown in this soil will still seek nutrients, more than are provided by the fertilisers and so send out a deeper and wider root system to draw in water in an effort to find the needed nutrients it lacks. This means that these plants become more water dependent and use more water than a plant in nutrient dense soil would need. This continual absorption of water in an effort to find nutrients causes the fruits or vegetables to swell to larger sizes, but this extra growth is still marred by lack of nutrition. Think of the large tomatoes, cucumbers, apples or oranges you may have purchased that tasted bland and had little flavour? Why is that? It is simply because the plant has grown in poor soils and so has produced foods swollen with water in an attempt to draw in nutrients. Water laden foods will taste exactly as expected, watery and bland. On the flip side high quality soils not exposed to fertilisers or other chemical sprays and enriched through compost and decaying matter, as nature has done for centuries, will be full of a wide spectrum of minerals, micro-organisms and earthworms. This

Nutrition's Playground

leads to a good layer of topsoil that retains an abundance of water and serves as a nutrient rich reservoir for plants to grow in.

If you were to purchase tomatoes, cucumbers, apples or oranges from a high quality, local, organic farm you may find the size of such produce is slightly smaller, but the depth of colour and richness of flavour more than compensate and the foods are much more satisfying because they are nutrient dense. Think about this. Smaller, more nutrient dense produce that satisfies more readily than conventional products. This sounds like a viable addition to managing excess weight by providing fewer calories with higher nutrient content and therefore satisfying appetite more quickly. Hopefully it is now clear that a tomato is not just a tomato. The farming and food management history will determine whether the product that is harvested is what nature intended as a nutrient rich tomato or whether it is merely a water filled skeleton of a tomato that is difficult to tell from the original just by looks alone. There are so many foods available today that serve as imposters to the nourishing, natural food that we should be eating, and as such do not deliver vibrant health. Without the knowledge of what to look for these imposters may never be identified and health may continue to elude us despite our best efforts.

The real purpose of this chapter is to expose the impostors in our food chain and seek out and describe the truly natural foods that will nourish us for generations. Only with the knowledge and understanding needed to identify and purchase the highest quality foods we can afford will we be able to shift ourselves up the optimal health spectrum away from a dependency on medication or synthetic supplementation to make up the shortfall in our diets. As the demand for these higher quality foods increases, farming and

Nutrition's Playground

food production will shift towards these methods to meet the demand and keep farms and businesses thriving.

Vibrant fruit and vegetables

We have already touched on some of the principles surrounding fruit and vegetable production. It is important to understand that although fruit and vegetables of differing quality can look similar, they are very different from a nutritional and taste perspective. First let's identify what should be minimised and avoided. Conventionally produced, dried, sweetened and crystallised fruit, fruit juice made from concentrate, tinned fruit in syrup, tinned vegetables or the minimal fruit pieces or concentrates used in snack foods and health bars. All these provide a nutrient poor source of calories and should be avoided. It must be remembered that fruit is rich in sugar and when there is little nutrition to go with the sugar found in fruits it carries little health benefit and upsets blood sugar balance which can lead to reactive eating and excessive insulin levels. Concentrated fruit juice is not a valid contributor to the 5 a day principle despite efforts to advertise this. It would not be unusual for a typical concentrated fruit juice to be sourced from conventional fruits grown in depleted, fertilised soils, having been sprayed with pesticides several times during their life cycle. These are then juiced in large industrial machines and pasteurised to kill any potential bacteria. The juice is then concentrated by boiling and evaporating the water in order to reduce the volume and make it cheaper to ship abroad. The concentrated juice will have lost many of its fragile nutrients by this point, but still retain the traces of industrial chemicals that were used in its production. Once received in the country of sale the concentrate is reconstituted with water and pasteurised again to ensure no further bacterial contamination, but to ensure it can be sold as a valid source of vitamin C it is common to then have synthetic vitamin C, ascorbic acid, added prior to packaging in the familiar tetra pack cartons. What is purchased and consumed is a far cry from the healthy, nutritious fruit advertised. This juice really is only sugar rich, flavoured water with pesticide residues, rather than a healthy food. It should not be considered a portion of fruit. It is not.

Conventionally produced, dried, sweetened fruit may still carry the fibre and retain more of the of the original product than fruit juice, but has had processed sugars added, it is industrially dried at temperatures which do not cook the food, but still destroy fragile easily oxidised nutrients like vitamin C. The pesticide residues will also still be present in these products. Tinned fruit and vegetables may provide a longer lasting product but are often of lower quality to begin with, which is why they are tinned and not sold as fresh, fruit and vegetables. They would not make the strict standards set for retail as class A produce. So they get tinned and sold under the guise of a beautiful picture on the tin that does not really represent what is inside. Fruits are always preserved in sugary syrup or in a fruit concentrate or fruit juice. Interestingly the health conscious buyer may feel the tinned fruit in fruit juice is much healthier than one in syrup. This is another marketing pretence as they are little better. The juices used are typically grape, apple or pear. These three are chosen because they are the fruits with the highest fructose content in nature and as such will have the highest sweetness levels. Fructose is a sugar that causes negative effects to the liver and upsets blood triglycerides or cholesterol levels. It is not a better option to have a fructose rich juice or syrup. More sugar from depleted fruits is about as beneficial as sugar drawn from depleted sugar beet or sugar cane. It all ultimately comes from plants, sugar is sugar.

Nutrition's Playground

The ideal fruit and vegetables are those grown in living soils rich in a wide spectrum of minerals, micro-organisms and earthworms without the use of fertilisers, pesticides, herbicides or fungicides. A minimum of organic standard farming would be desirable, but biodynamic farmed food is an even better standard. Fruit and vegetables should be sourced as local as possible to reduce food miles and transportation that always introduces pollution. The further away they are transported the earlier the produce will be picked before it has ripened which also serves to decrease the nutrient content. Finally fruit and vegetables should ideally be eaten in season as this will help to optimise nutrient levels. Eating in season will encourage a varied intake throughout the year as produce moves into and out of season. Other types and varieties of fruits and vegetables will be tried and enjoyed. Trying to eat produce in this way will likely introduce some challenges. It will be difficult to eat fruit and vegetables that tick all these criteria when the supermarket is relied upon to supply the food. Whilst organic produce is often available it is common place to find it has been sourced from another country and travelled many food miles and as a result has been picked unripe and out of season. If you know what fruit and vegetables are in season you will become aware that the supermarkets do increase their stocks of the 'in season' produce at these times of year and often the price goes down slightly because they are in plentiful supply. Sometimes this may be the only time that produce is sourced from the country it is bought in, but there is still no guarantee it is local and it may still have been transported several hundred miles. In order to buy organic, local and seasonal fresh fruit and vegetables it is best to buy from a local fruit and vegetable box delivery scheme or to visit a local farm shop and only buy their own produce that meets these standards. This has become so much more common in the UK and there is an excellent network of farm shops and box schemes around the country.

Nutrition's Playground

Delicious dairy produce

Dairy is a huge industry in the UK with only a handful of large companies controlling the majority of milk in the country. The concerns around pasteurisation and poor quality milk were discussed in an earlier chapter and the ideal was identified as being organic, grass fed, unprocessed, fresh raw milk. Just to clarify lets be 100% clear on what to avoid and what to seek. Pasteurised, homogenised, industrial farmed milk, especially skimmed and semi skimmed, low fat yogurts of all types, standard cheese, cream or soured cream and industrial farmed butter should all be avoided. These products come from milk that has been sourced mostly from large scale farms and dairies where the cattle live in cramped conditions, are fed grains and other cattle feed such as soya, citrus peel, extruded grains and bakery waste and are usually dosed with routine antibiotics in their feed. They are usually high milk yield breeds, like Holstein, which produce a large volume of lower quality milk which has lower nutrient density. The cattle are often milked for as long and as often as possible. This means they may be impregnated and calf too close together to allow the cow to rebuild her reserves before she is placed back on the milking round. This leads to stress and depletion of the quality of the milk. Any dairy produce made from this type of low quality milk cannot be made healthy no matter what man adds or does to process it. Usually any processing the milk goes through, especially pasteurisation and homogenisation further destroys any goodness that was there. The vast majority of milk, cheese and yoghurt sold in supermarkets fall into this category.

If you search carefully there are a few slightly higher quality products that can serve as a stepping stone towards consuming the ideal dairy products. These would be whole milk products that come from organic farms particularly

Nutrition's Playground

yoghurt, butter and cheeses. Organic whole milk, whilst it comes from healthier cows, has in most cases still been pasteurised and homogenised. This is still undesirable. If organic milk that has only been pasteurised and has not undergone homogenisation is available, then this is a better option and will serve as a transition to better milk. Many of the beneficial nutrients found in milk are either in the fat or need the fat to help assimilate the nutrients into our bodies, so always seek whole milk and dairy products. The low fat products usually taste bland and lose their texture and consistency so in the case of yoghurt and cream cheeses they add starches and thickeners to try and regain the lost properties and to prevent them being too watery.

It is very likely that to buy the best dairy products will require a trip to a farm shop or a farmers market. Whilst there are only a limited number of suppliers of high quality, unpasteurised dairy in the United Kingdom, it is worth the effort to purchase and consume this food where possible. Jersey and Guernsey pure bred herds produce the highest quality milk as they produce a much lower volume of milk with a more significant volume of cream and nutrients. The proteins in the milk from these two breeds has been shown to be more favourable for the human gut as well and is less likely to cause allergies than the typical Holstein breeds. It is important that the cattle are grass fed as much as possible throughout the year and that the farmer prepares natural feed such as silage or hay to feed the cattle during the winter months when it becomes too cold and damp to let the herd graze on pasture. If unpasteurised milk of these standards cannot be found, but a supplier of organic, pasteurised, grass fed, Jersey or Guernsey milk and dairy can be found this will be the next best option. High quality dairy can make an excellent addition to the diet, especially in young and growing children, all the way through to adulthood, where it provides essential nutrients. Whilst adults do not have such a vital need for milk it is still a highly nutritious and valuable food source and should be encouraged where it is possible to buy better quality sources.

Mouth-watering meat and poultry

The meat and poultry industry is perhaps fraught with more undesirable and bad practises that reduce the quality of the final products than almost any other industry. This means that the consumer needs to be informed and vigilant about which products they choose to buy. These bad practises have been introduced in many cases to make the overall meat rearing and management process cheaper or faster. An example of this is that in post war Europe it would typically take about 4-5 years to grow a cow large enough for slaughter, whereas today in many cases this can be achieved in less than 18 months. Many factors have contributed to this significantly quicker production, from carefully selected breeding to weed out any slower growing genetics, the development of what is referred to as double muscled cows and the predominance of grain based, low quality feeds that replace large amounts of the diet. The acidic grains are considerably more potent as weight gaining fodder than grass. They do, however, produce cattle that have much higher levels of stored body fat than cattle reared on grass, but this has little effect on the price the meat is sold for, which in many cases is on the weight of product. So the modern beef farmer can raise selectively bred cattle to become larger and fatter in a third of the time today than was possible 50-60 years ago. This enables a higher turnover of stock to ensure that business is more profitable and the butchers or supermarkets that sell this meat can do so at a lower price. Prices are so low on some meat products that we have become deceptively conditioned into what an appropriate price to pay for our meat produce actually is. Ground minced

Nutrition's Playground

beef; cheap burgers and meat pies often have little quality worth talking about, but are highly affordable.

The poultry industry, particularly chicken, has received a lot of media coverage in recent years over the way in which vast amount of birds are reared in record time to maintain our demand for this 'lower' fat bird. A typical barn reared chick is now intensively grown and ready for slaughter in only 39 days, if it survives the brutal world of industrial chicken farming. In 1998 the UK broiler chicken industry hatched 793.4 million chicks with 745.6 million birds reaching the slaughterhouse amassing over £2 billion in sales. Approximately 90% of all chickens grown in the UK are reared within the standard intensively reared system. Despite the information regarding how these chickens are reared being freely available today, intensively reared chicken is still a buoyant industry. The standard intensive poultry system can be outlined as follows:

- Chicks at 1 day old are placed in barns with no outdoor access for the full 39 day rearing period

- Barn is completely bare except for feeding and drinking pots

- 23 hours a day of bright fluorescent bulbs ensure that chickens are encouraged to feed as much as possible

- First mortalities begin to happen within the first week

- The barns are only cleared out after the full 39 days, meaning the chickens live in their own excrement

Nutrition's Playground

- It is common for birds resting on the ground to get hock burns on their legs from the potent ammonia from their excrement

- Boredom sets in, with nothing to do or generate interest, birds often fight and peck at each other

- Halfway through the experience the lights are dimmed for 4 hours a day to allow rest

- As the chickens grow there is less and less space for them

- to move around -typical EU stocking density is 17-20 birds per square metre
- Such rapid growth in body weight, with little ability to move around leads to birds who are too weak to carry such bulk and approximately 25% of birds are found to develop lameness and leg deformities

- Millions of birds die from heart failure each year – the mortality rates amongst intensively reared birds is seven times as much as slow growing egg laying hens

- Intensively reared chickens spend nearly 75% of their time sitting compared to only 30% in normal free range birds

- Ammonia concentrations in the air can become so toxic that they cause lung irritation, inflammation and lead to disease

- Growing temperatures in the poorly ventilated barns lead to heat stress and aggravation of the birds

Nutrition's Playground

- A few days prior to slaughter the birds are deprived of food and water to ensure their intestinal contents are empty to make the process easier to manage

These conditions are only ever going to rear distressed, unhealthy, overweight birds that will never provide humans with valuable nutrition. However, with the ridiculously low prices that these birds are sold for it seems that many are willing to push this knowledge to the back of their minds and purchase this type of chicken anyway. This is a short term decision. Whilst money is saved initially by purchasing such cheap chicken and other low cost foods, in the long term as health declines, low quality food choices, the cost of health care and diminished quality of life demand the debt be repaid.

In today's meat and poultry market grass fed, free range, organic produce does fetch a higher price, but it has taken some time for the general public to appreciate that it is a higher quality product that has had much more work and effort put into it. Still the higher prices tend to be a barrier for many people who deem it outside their price range. So what is it that makes good quality meat worth the additional investment? Buying organic meat ensures that the animals will be reared to decent ethical standards and that in many cases the animals will get to live outdoors when the weather is appropriate Though do look for other indicators of this such as 'free range', or 'grass fed' just to be sure. Organic will also guarantee that there has been no routine use of antibiotics in the animal feed and they will not be exposed to pesticides, herbicides or fertilisers, either on the land they roam or in any feed they are given. This is important. Regular use of antibiotics allows disease resistant strains of bacteria to develop in the guts of the ruminant animals like cows and sheep. These very damaging pathogenic bacteria can make their way easily into the food chain, even in non meat products because manure is used to fertilise the land and plants.

Destructive bacteria, like E Coli H157, have killed hospitalised and sickened thousands of people. E Coli began its life as a mutated strain of bacteria growing in the digestive tracts of unhealthy, intensively reared cattle eating grain and cheap feeds with antibiotics added to try and stop them getting sick. The bacteria got out and human illness is the result. Animals that live outdoors also get the freedom to roam and be active as animals should be. It has been well proven that human beings should be active as part of a healthy lifestyle. This is a basic necessity for animals too. They should not be cooped up inside a barn or feedlot as this creates stress and leads to diminished levels of health. Roaming outdoors eating grass, foraging around trees, bushes and hedges is much more enjoyable and relaxing for the animals and adds to their health and well being. This will greatly improve the quality of the end product we eat, whether that is meat, dairy, poultry or eggs.

Organic, free range animals have been found to have naturally lower fat stored on their frame because they are active and they eat foods they were designed to eat. On the other hand cattle, sheep or chicken fed lots of grains and cheep feeds become much fatter and their meat lacks certain nutrients that are drawn from the grass and the outdoor life. Fats soluble nutrients like vitamins A, D and K2 and anti-carcinogenic compounds like conjugated linolenic acid (CLA) are only found in significant levels in grass fed animals. Good quality farms will allow more time for their animals to reach an optimal weight for slaughter, sometimes more than twice as long, ensuring that they lead a natural, stress free, healthy life along the way. Animals raised as close to how Mother Nature intended will develop optimal health which will then

214

Nutrition's Playground

be passed on up the food chain and benefit us. It is ludicrous to think that animals raised in artificial, intensive systems that are ultimately unhealthy can then serve to make us healthy! Health has to be passed up the food chain. You cannot draw health from that which is unhealthy or, as one old farmer said, "ya cain't give what ya ain't got any more'n ya can go back to where you've never bin!"

Satisfying grains and pulses

Grains and pulses have been considered the staff of life or staple foods for generations. In almost every culture around the world, grains and/or beans have formed part of the diet as far back as recorded history can inform us. Wheat was discussed in an earlier chapter and we know the wheat grown today is not the same as that grown traditionally. Wheat has been selectively bred, it is usually mono cropped in depleted soils, it is subject to pesticide and herbicide sprays, it is often ground into white flour with the husk and the nutritious germ removed leaving behind the empty carbohydrate component. This flour is made into all kinds of goods and products from pastries and bread to gravy granules, sweeteners and bulking agents. Whilst wheat is one of the major grains grown and utilised throughout the world, there are two others that also serve as staple foods, rice and maize (corn). The primary grown bean in the world is the soya bean. The two most widely grown genetically modified crops are maize and soya beans. Grains, beans and pulses serve as staple foods in the diet of over 4 billion people in the world and so have an influence perhaps more than any other food on our health and metabolism. This means that we not only have to learn sources we avoid and what we seek, but we also need to know how to best prepare and utilise these food stuffs effectively.

Nutrition's Playground

We must avoid all sources of genetically modified grains, especially soya and maize. The law does not require food labels to identify if a source of GM soya or maize has been used in the manufacture of a product. Maize and soya are used in breads, cakes, pastries, sauces, ice cream, wheat free foods, crisps, nachos, tortillas, pizza, gravy granules, confectionery, chocolate, cereal bars, biscuits, tofu, soya milk, vegetarian meat alternatives and many other processed food products. None of these conventional products are required to inform you they have been manufactured from a GM crop. There is only one certain answer to this dilemma, which is to buy organic. European organic standards do not allow the use of any GM materials in foodstuffs that are certified organic. Buying organic will also rule out the contamination of these foods with pesticide and herbicide residues. As a general rule we should avoid where possible any refined, non organic, grains and pulses or their derivatives, especially those used in the manufacture of processed, convenience foods such as those listed above. In many cases these will not provide optimal health and will increase the stress and toxic load upon the body.

As has been preached for some time now we should really emphasise using the whole grain products, pulses and beans where possible. These should also be drawn from organic sources and if you can determine the origin, ideally as local as possible. In many cases dried beans and pulses will be imported from other countries. In such cases buying organic and fair-trade will at least ensure a minimum standard of quality and aid the farmer in receiving a certain minimum wage for his/her efforts. When it comes to grains it may be wise to shift away from our reliance on wheat as the primary grain. Wheat grown today is a hybrid species that has been developed to cope with the harsh mechanised bread making process. Most wheat is grown as part of mono-cropping systems in depleted soils with regular use of nitrogen and other fertilisers and typical spraying of pesticides and herbicides. Wheat is often stored prior to milling and distribution in large grain silos where the tendency to mould and mildew growth is prevented with further sprays and chemicals. These all end up in the final product, the flour we eat. Using more traditional varieties such as spelt, rye and buck wheat (not of the wheat family despite the name) will prove more nutritious and digestible compared to typical modern wheat, especially if they are organically grown. It is also becoming more common to be able to purchase organically grown whole grains before they are milled. This will retain the greatest nutrient density because as soon as the grains are milled, even if they are organic, the nutrients are no longer protected by the outer husk and they begin to degrade and oxidise.

It is best that grains and pulses are soaked in slightly acidic, lukewarm water for some time prior to use. This is most easily done overnight in preparation for the next day's food and meals. This pre-digests the grains, beans, lentils or chickpeas and makes the nutrients more bioavailable to us and is how these foods were traditionally prepared for centuries prior to modern convenience foods becoming so readily available. Certain beans and legumes may even require 2 days of soaking to neutralise the natural toxins contained within. There are certain products available today made from soaked or sprouted grains, such as organic sourdough and sprouted grain breads; these are delicious and nutritious food products that still provide the convenience of not needing to make your own bread.

Sumptuous seafood

Seafood used to be a fairly simple industry when it came down to quality. The fresher the catch the more likely it was

Nutrition's Playground

that the fish or shellfish would have been of good quality because all fish was caught wild from oceans and rivers. Today this has drastically changed. Concerns regarding over fishing the natural reserves available in the seas has led to the development of fish farming. This is where vast populations of fish are grown in cramped conditions in large tanks, artificial lakes, or large pens in the sea. They are fed a regular stream of processed fish food to speed up the growth of the fish in order to maximise both size and time it takes until the fish are ready to eat. This intensive farming system is not unlike the typical barn production of standard chicken, only it is in water. There can literally be thousands of fish farmed in relatively small space, with no great distance to move or swim. They live in the same water that they excrete in for considerable periods of their short life where the cramped, polluted conditions typically lead to disease and degeneration of the fish. The fish farming industry does not currently have the needed regulations to ensure the welfare and quality of the fish beyond ensuring they are fit for human consumption. Needless to say in most cases farmed fish should be minimised and even avoided in the diet.

In the case of fish, buying organic is not as sensible an option as it is with many other food categories. This is because organic fish are still farmed fish! The only way in which the standards laid down by organic regulations can be guaranteed is to farm the fish. The stocking densities are not as high and the feed is of course sourced organically, but nonetheless it is still farmed fish. Farmed organic fish may serve as an appropriate transitional change to purchasing the best quality fish. The best fish to buy are those that have been reared by Mother Nature herself and hence should be wild caught ocean going or river fish. These fish have been able to swim freely through different environments and habitats and eat a much wider variety of food with greater nutrient density. These factors lead to stronger, healthier fish than a typical fish farm can produce.

The problem as far a large scale supermarkets are concerned is that wild caught ocean going fish have unpredictable supplies, whereas fish farming can produce to demand. This means that there are few wild fish sold in supermarkets today. It is likely that local fishmongers will sell a wider range of ocean caught fish, but even then there will still be a plentiful supply of farmed fish. Careful shopping is needed in purchasing seafood which is an essential contributor to good health. In the studies that Weston A. Price made of healthy, indigenous cultures he found that seafood served as a backbone in every diet where eating fish was possible due to geographical location. It was prized for its health promoting properties. A variety of white and oily fish with the inclusion of shellfish on occasion should be included where the quality of the fish can be guaranteed. In areas where it is too difficult to get high quality fish it is possible to draw on the needed nutrients through purchasing high quality fish oils, such as cod liver oil. Look for oils made from wild fish that have not been chemically cleaned and deodorised and contain naturally occurring vitamin A and D in a ratio of 5 to 1.

Nutritious natural sweeteners

There are many foods and compounds used to sweeten food today, the large majority of which should be avoided if good health and weight loss is the goal. Refined castor, granulated, demerera and other brown sugars should be completely avoided. These sweeteners are only a shell of the naturally occurring compounds from which they originated. They contain empty calories with no vitamins and minerals, the digestion of which steal nutrients and devitalises our resources. Syrups such as golden syrup, treacle, agave, fruit

Nutrition's Playground

concentrates and high fructose syrups should also be expressly avoided. These are also highly concentrated, devitalised sources of simple carbohydrates that will only serve to damage the body, upset blood sugar and disrupt human metabolism. Artificial sweeteners such as aspartame, acesulfame K, saccharin and sucralose are all synthetic chemicals which have considerable risks associated with their regular consumption. The risks run from simple symptoms such as muscular aching and mental fogginess all the way through to damaged brain cells and dementia. Whilst these more severe symptoms affect only a minority of people, it isn't worth the risk to find out whether you are one who will suffer or not.

Some sweeteners have had less processing and therefore still retain some natural goodness that may assist in their assimilation. Organic maple syrup, rapadura and unheated, unfiltered honey can offer an element of sweetness when required whilst still offering nutrients that can benefit the body. Maple syrup and rapadura, which is dehydrated cane sugar juice, still retain some of the needed minerals that can assist the body. Raw honey retains minerals, enzymes, pollen and propolis that can assist in maintaining health in conjunction with our natural foods. However, it must still be remembered that whilst each of these are better than most refined sweeteners, large amounts of each will still upset blood sugars. They should be used occasionally in moderation. The primary step towards good health in relation to sweeteners is to wean yourself off too many sweet foods and condition your taste buds over 2 - 4 weeks to adjust to lower levels of sweetness. Once this has been done the drive to seek sweet foods is somewhat diminished and when sweet foods are eaten they quickly become unpalatable so that less will be eaten in any one go.

Nutrition's Playground

Beautiful beverages

There are so many different types of fluids to drink it can be difficult to know what is healthy and what is not. Fruit juice is perhaps one category that is considered to be healthy and, in fact, one of our 5 a day. This is not true in most cases. Conventional fruit juice made from concentrates, squeezed fruit juices not from concentrate and fruit flavoured cordials all offer a significant dose of sugar. In all cases these drinks will have lost considerable nutrients through their processing and packaging. They are also quickly ingested and absorbed and so taken on their own will upset blood sugar and imbalance energy metabolism. They will also provide a concentrated source of agricultural chemicals that are retained from the original fruit. Whilst purchasing organic fruit juices is an improvement, the reality is that nutrients will still have oxidised and been lost, leaving behind a sweet, sugary drink. If fruit juice is to impart valuable nutrition, it is best to squeeze or juice fresh, organic fruit and drink it within a relatively short time to ensure that the nutrients are retained. Exposure to light and air will allow for nutrient losses to occur. The same concerns apply to vegetable juice of commercial and organic origin. The best option is to juice your own organic vegetables and drink them within a relatively short time.

Tea and coffee are both well recognised stimulants with a whole concoction of chemicals contained within. Caffeine, tannin, pesticide residues and other chemicals all serve to challenge the body every time a cup is consumed. Indeed these drinks do serve to pick up the metabolism briefly, but it is not as a result of improving energy resources that this occurs. Caffeine stimulates the adrenal glands, which in turn release hormones that encourage the body to release energy from its own reserves. Once the effect wears off the individual is left with slightly lower energy and depleted reserves than they had before the cup of tea or coffee was consumed. This increases the likelihood of a repeat cup being consumed. This leads to dependency and addiction, which is common in those who drink tea and coffee. Where possible efforts should be put in place to reduce and avoid tea and coffee consumption. There are a variety of organic herbal teas available today that can provide an alternative hot beverage that is more nourishing to the body. However, a word of caution is required regarding herbal teas. Herbs have been used as a form of medicine for generations and teas composed of medicinal herbs can exert considerable effects on the body. Take some time to determine the effects of the herbs in the teas you seek to drink and choose wisely for your needs. It may be best to have 2 or 3 different herbal teas that serve different purposes and to select rather than just by flavour, but on what effect the tea will have based on current needs. Then a refreshing hot drink can be enjoyed and the body can be sustained and kept healthy in the process.

Perhaps one of the biggest beverage markets is that of soft drinks. Some of the most profitable companies in the world are soft drinks manufacturers. In 2008 the UK soft drinks market was valued at over £13 billion with more than 13,905 million litres consumed. Consumption of this volume works out at approximately 228 litres per person per year, with almost 42% of the market or 100 litres of the total coming from carbonated soft drinks! This indicates that the average person in the UK consumes a litre of carbonated soft drinks every 3.6 days, or about 2 litres per week. It seems that here in the UK we have a different type of drinking problem. Carbonated soft drinks can wreak havoc on the human body when consumed regularly over time. There is little nutrition, if any, found in modern soft drinks. They are often very high in sugar, which rarely comes from sugar cane or beet, but is usually derived from glucose syrup or high fructose corn

Nutrition's Playground

syrups. These sweet syrups are likely to have been made from genetically modified corn and are enzymatically altered to have a higher than natural fructose content. This makes them sweeter than standard syrups or sugars and so saves the manufacturers a little money as less is required. The problem is that high fructose sugars have been found to really imbalance normal blood metabolism. Fructose has been found to disturb normal mineral balance in the blood particularly that of calcium, increasing urinary outputs. Whilst fructose does not have a great effect on blood insulin levels, it does increase the formation of blood triglycerides, but does not increase their removal from the blood into fat tissues. This type of blood fat, a triglyceride, has recently been reconfirmed as having links with heart disease and elevated cholesterol levels. Many carbonated soft drinks, especially colas are also rich in phosphoric acid, an additive used to acidify beverages and provide a tangy, slightly sour taste. However, this also has an acidifying effect on the blood which has to be counterbalanced. Changing the pH of the blood has an effect on the whole metabolism of the body. Whilst the effects on pH from soft drinks may only be small it can lead over time to decreasing health. Some studies have shown that regular carbonated soft drink consumption may negatively affect bone density as the body releases calcium from the bones to buffer the acidifying effect.

If high fructose syrups and phosphoric acid are not enough, most soft drinks also have potent colours, chemical flavourings and sweeteners like aspartame and acesulfame K. As previously mentioned there is little in a modern carbonated soft drink that is beneficial to the body. They really should be minimised or avoided where possible.

Once again tradition provides an alternative option for the modern soft drink that can provide some health benefits at the same time as an enjoyable and refreshing drink. Before technology developed the ability to force carbon dioxide under pressure into beverages to carbonate the drink, soft drinks were naturally brewed and fermented. The fermentation process carbonated the drink and gave it the fizz that adds to the enjoyment of the finished product. However, this process of lacto-fermentation takes time and patience, which is not a trait most modern businesses have. Time is money in today's world. So tradition has been pushed aside in the search for money and soft drinks are made quickly from cheap, destructive ingredients.

Lacto-fermentation is the process of using the good bacteria that naturally occur in milk to ferment a food or in this case a beverage. Whilst there are many flavours and types of lacto-fermented drink a relatively simple and widely enjoyed option is to brew some traditional mild lemon ginger ale. Once allowed an appropriate fermentation time and then chilled in the fridge it makes for a truly refreshing drink that has minimal sugar, is rich in minerals and has a healthy dose of beneficial bacteria to support and maintain gut flora.

Although this may not sound as exciting, the most important beverage for us to consume is water. However, even this simple, life sustaining drink is fraught with some modern pitfalls. Tap water is treated today with a host of chemicals to cleanse and purify and in some cases even to mass medicate the population. It is standard practise for tap water to have added chlorine which kills most bacteria to make the water safe to drink. Whilst we are told the levels are very small and safe for human consumption, over a lifetime this can chip away at our health. Although not widespread in the UK water fluoridation does occur in some regions of the country. The primary justification for adding fluoride, one of the more toxic substances known to man, to the water supply is that there are some indications that fluoride may prevent dental

Nutrition's Playground

decay. Rather than give the public the choice of how they prevent dental decay some water boards have taken that decision without informing the public and fluoridate the water any way.

The US has much more widespread water fluoridation, whereas in the UK only 9% of the population live in areas with artificially fluoridated water. Fluoride is a very reactive substance that has a strong affinity for calcium and so is often found in the form of calcium fluoride. The theory is that ingested fluoride ultimately bonds with the calcium that makes up the teeth, strengthening the enamel and creating a resistance to decay. Despite these apparent benefits, stained and mottled teeth as a result of fluorosis are much higher in areas where water is fluoridated. Interestingly the number of dentists and the average spend per person on dental health is also higher in the regions of the UK where fluoride is added to water when compared to non-fluoridated regions. This does not offer much support to the theory of cavity protection. There are even some possible links of fluoride in the drinking water and increased rates of bone cancer and the occurrence of osteoporosis.

The best way to get around this is, at the very least, to filter your tap water using a typical carbon filter. This helps to remove chlorine, fluoride and any heavy metals that may be in your drinking supply such as aluminium, copper and lead. Whilst this will never be perfect, it is much better than drinking tap water direct. Bottled water is not the answer either in most cases, especially since most water is packaged in plastic bottles. The water may be pure and rich in minerals when drawn from the source, but after weeks and months in a bottle stored in warm conditions, the plastic chemicals can leach into the water increasing the levels of xenoestrogens. These are oestrogen mimicking compounds that can disrupt hormone balance and human function. If the water is mineral rich, over 300mg dissolved solids, and is bottled in glass, then it is likely to be a good reliable source of quality drinking water.

Quality Counts

Whilst this has not been an exhaustive discussion on the foods to avoid and the foods to seek, it has dealt with the major food and beverage categories. We must shift our perception away from the concept that all fruit is fruit and bread is bread. It is clear that apple juice squeezed and pasteurised from standard pesticide laden fruit shipped in from abroad and the product of more than one country is not the same as eating a locally produced organic apple in the height of apple season. White bread made from intensively grown, refined wheat flour, vegetable oils, soya flour, preservatives and mould inhibitors is not the same as eating whole grain, organic sourdough bread made from locally produced organic wheat, filtered water, unprocessed salt and nothing else. When these differences are considered honestly and fairly it is clear that food quality really counts. It does make a difference to us, both nutritionally and in regards to our health, where we choose to purchase our food and what quality of food we are willing to invest in. Often the higher prices for food items of better quality is the reason used to continue to justify the purchase of lower quality foods. Where finances are genuinely tight this is understandable. However, it is important to start somewhere. Excuses always seem to immobilise us and prevent change.

I have worked with people over the years who complained about the cost of better food being a burden, yet they still socialised and spent considerable amounts of money on alcohol on a Friday and Saturday night. Some said they couldn't afford better food yet they spent money regularly on

Nutrition's Playground

buying lunch during their working day and eating out two or three nights a week. Some said it was a matter of principle they were not prepared to pay out for higher priced foods, yet at home they have all the latest branded gadgets and technology. Some said it wasn't worth paying the extra money for the same food that could be purchased cheaper, yet the clothing they wore was always expensive branded items that could be purchased cheaper elsewhere if they stopped worrying about the brand name. What we are prepared to invest in our food will greatly depend on where food comes in our hierarchy of values. If a nice car, technical gadgets, socialising, top clothing and other things far exceed the importance of buying natural, wholesome foods it is unlikely that increased investment will be spared to purchase these more nutritious options. If food sits lower down the pecking order of priorities, only money left over once each higher priority has had its piece of the monthly income can then be invested into food shopping. It would be ridiculous to expect people to stop doing or buying everything else in life that they enjoy just so they can afford to purchase good food, but it is highly likely that some small compromises can be identified. Instead of spending £40 on a night out, save £5 and only spend £35 and then you will be able to buy all your fruit and vegetables organically with the money spared. Instead of buying the best brands on all clothes, perhaps on items such as socks and plain tops that are not the primary item, but supportive of the overall outfit, money can be saved that could be invested into better food. When food becomes a higher priority there will always be a solution to finding the extra finance to cover the costs.

It may take time to gradually work through different elements of your routine diet and item by item start changing the quality of what is eaten. Tastes, textures and preferences need to adjust as well as the budget. Soon small changes, like drinking herbal instead of regular tea, become the norm and

Nutrition's Playground

don't seem like a challenge any more. Once a change feels part of the routine it is much easier to make another change in the right direction until that feels normal. It is very easy to look at the diet you are eating and the quality food you would like to be eating and to see such a vast difference that the change seems beyond you. This can lead to inaction because it appears that it is not worth trying because you are likely to fail. Let me assure you it is always worth trying, no matter how big the task seems. There is always a way to make a difference. You just need to believe it is possible first. The next chapters of the book will explore this area of making a change to our beliefs about food and eating to fuel a change in dietary choices.

Perhaps one of the most important lessons that can be learned about food is that quality counts, quality counts, quality really counts! It is our basic right to have access to food that will keep us healthy and vibrant throughout our lives. Demand that right in your life and make it happen.

Nutrition's Playground

Step 9: Act or React

It is important to consider how best to make the transition towards a nutrient dense, traditional, whole food diet. In the modern world with the mass media constantly providing an outlet for food marketing and mixed messages about what is nutritious and beneficial to eat, it can be difficult to turn an initial desire to make a change into a lifelong habit. I wonder how many well intentioned efforts to lose weight or eat a healthier diet have been scuppered by an impulse to buy some quick, cheap food advertised or being sold in the high street or supermarket? I wonder how many people slip off the straight and narrow path to a healthy nutritious lifestyle because of the constant advertising bombarding us through television or radio every day to purchase fast foods and other junk? I wonder how many have pledged to eat a healthy, balanced diet, but somewhere hidden in the kitchen is a favourite junk food snack, like chocolate or ice cream, just in case they need a nibble to hold them through? I wonder how many people have justified that others living in the house won't change, so they still buy lower quality foods to feed the others, whilst they alienate themselves with a healthier diet. This becomes a point of contention or ridicule and, as a result, they break their resolve. Why is it so difficult to make changes to the way we eat?

The 2010 Fortune 500 list of the most financially successful companies in the USA has rated Wal-mart as number one with annual revenues of over $408 billion and profits of $14.3 billion. That is an annual turnover larger than the national budget of many countries around the world. Wal-mart own

Nutrition's Playground

the supermarket chain Asda in the UK. The following table shows a list of companies that also retail in the food and drink markets of the world and who made the 2010 top 500.

Company	Food Brands	Revenues	Profits
Proctor and Gamble	Pringles	$79 billion	$13 billion
Costco wholesale	Kirkland	$71 billion	$1 billion
Pepsi Co	Pepsi, Frito Lay, Doritos, Tropicana, Quaker, Gatorade	$43 billion	$6 billion
Kraft foods	Cadbury, Capri-sun, Dentyne, Halls, Kenco, Kool Aid, Maxwell House, Oreo, Philadelphia, Ritz, Toblerone	$40 billion	$3 billion
Coca Cola	Fanta, Sprite, Lilt, Oasis, Schweppes, Kia-Ora, 5 Alive, Minute Maid, Powerade, Relentless, Malvern	$31 billion	$7 billion
Tyson Foods	Meat products	$27 billion	
McDonalds	Fast foods	$23 billion	$4.5 billion

Nutrition's Playground

Company	Food Brands	Revenues	Profits
Sara Lee	Douwe Egberts, Prima, Sara Lee, Brylcreem, Sanex, Ambi-pur,	$12 billion	$360 million
Kellogg's	Cornflakes, Bran flakes, All bran, Coco pops, Frosties, Optivita, Fruit Winders, Special K, Pop tarts, Nutri-grain	$12.6 billion	$1.2 billion
Dean Foods	Meadow Gold, Rachel's	$11 billion	$240 million
Heinz	Lea & Perrins, Weight Watchers, TGI Fridays	$10 billion	$920 million
Starbucks	Coffee, snack foods	$9 billion	$390 million
Dr Pepper	Dr Pepper	$5.5 billion	$555 million

There are vast sums of money being generated by many of these food and beverage companies, with enormous profit margins in the majority of cases. This allows for significant investment in advertising, sponsorship and media campaigns to increase brand awareness and to sell their products in every possible outlet. The quality of the vast majority of the products sold by these companies is of average to poor quality when compared to the standard of food needed for optimal health, as identified in the previous chapter. The influence and corporate power displayed by these financial

Nutrition's Playground

giants can be either inspiring or daunting depending which side of the fence you sit on. The brands and products they sell have become so influential that in many cases they have become weaved into the very fabric of life and affect our daily routines and lifestyle. How then do we move ourselves beyond their mighty influence to be able to introduce nutrient dense, natural foods into our diet?

The more time and effort we spend imprinting our minds with the logo's, brands and products sold by large food manufacturing companies, the greater influence they are likely to have upon us. After all that is the aim of advertising, to create enough awareness of a company or product to affect our buying choices. If we can remove ourselves from that advertising influence, it is less likely that our buying choices or buying impulses will be affected in a 'weak' moment to purchase lower quality foods that will negatively affect our health. This is a fairly difficult step to take but an important one nonetheless. The majority of people spend most of their time in reaction to someone or something else. Usually when this is pointed out we tend not to believe it and in contrast prefer to believe that we direct our own destiny and that we choose to live the way we do. However, when a deeper study of this concept, and the many areas of life that are influenced by this concept, is made it soon becomes apparent that human beings are very reactionary.

Sense and delete

The human body is designed to receive vast amounts of information at any given moment in time. Think about the senses that we have been given. Sight, sound, smell, taste and touch all provide us with a myriad of different information every second of the day. Then our own inner thoughts that are constantly reviewing and relaying this information have their own constant chatter to add even more to this mix of relentless information. Science has estimated that through our different sensory channels we receive about 2 million pieces of information for every second of the day. That seems unbelievable, because we just can't process that amount of information. Well, at least our conscious mind cannot process that amount of information. Whilst reading this book your eyes are focused on processing the information on the page into a stream of thought that may likely be occupying the majority of your conscious mind. However, if you stop and heighten your other senses you may realise that there are other stimuli that your were not paying attention too. What sounds can you hear? Perhaps other people, traffic, birds, television or even your own breathing can be clearly heard but you hadn't noticed until right now when it was brought to your conscious awareness. Are there any smells? Is there anything in your peripheral vision to add to the words on the page that you are reading now? What taste is in your mouth right now? What is in contact with your skin right now and what information is it providing about pressure, temperature and texture? What position are your arms and legs in? All of this information has just been brought back into your conscious awareness by the very fact that you were instructed to think about it though the words written on this page. All this sensory information was occurring previously to being made consciously aware and will continue to occur even when your conscious mind is not paying attention again.

Your subconscious mind is processing all of this information and much more all of the time whether your conscious mind is paying attention or not. Your brain is receiving about 2 million pieces of information per second, but it is not retaining 2 million pieces of information. The subconscious mind has to determine what information it should retain and hold onto and what information is less important and therefore it can delete. The brain chooses to retain just over a

Nutrition's Playground

hundred pieces of information every second from the vast sea of data that is constantly overwhelming us from the outside world. Yet even this volume of information every second is too much for your conscious mind to remain focused on and so our subconscious mind manages and controls what should be done with all this other information, determining whether any reaction needs to occur for our well being, safety or in maintaining balance.

Think about it

Just because we think something does not mean that we will act upon it. Food manufacturers and the world of advertising have developed very powerful systems for increasing their influence on our subconscious minds and therefore the chances that our conscious minds will register this data and generate thoughts sufficiently that we are more likely to act upon it. The more often certain thoughts pervade the arena of the mind the more likely it is that these thoughts will begin to have influence on us. Thought alone is not a very strong motivator to action, but thought coupled with an emotional response becomes a powerful force that is more persuasive and will usually lead to a response.

Think of a child at night whose thoughts have convinced them that there is something in the darkness of the room which in turn fuels fear to build up in conjunction with these thoughts. It is not long before that child will be crying or calling for their parents who then need to play to their logical mind to convince the child that their thoughts are misplaced and there is no need to have the fearful emotions. Consider a car salesman who is trying to get you beyond your thoughts that a new car would be nice. He is likely to go with you for a test drive so you can experience the feelings the car stirs up. Whilst on the journey he may ask questions like how you would feel on a hot summer's day driving with the soft top down and the wind rushing by. The salesman is trying to get you emotionally involved with the car because it is more likely that you will purchase when you become emotionally attached to it. Just like the scared child whose heightened emotions caused it to yell out for its parents, an adult who becomes emotionally attached to a product, like a car, is more likely to act and purchase that particular product.

The truth is that our thoughts lead to emotions which in turn are a powerful driving force for action. The actions we choose to engage in will have a significant impact on the results and outcomes that we are able to achieve. There is little that a human being can do without thinking about it first. It is true we have a number of reflexes that serve to protect us and respond with virtually no prior thought, such as pulling our hand off a hot object. Even the simple process of walking requires that we start with a thought from the conscious mind. We may have been thinking about some food that we might like to eat which sets in motion the intent to go to the kitchen. The thought of ice cream, crisps or a bar of chocolate sets off a series of past experiences in our mind where these foods created pleasure when eaten and in this moment that positive feeling is a powerful motivating force. The subconscious mind then takes over the control of the many muscles involved in driving the mechanics of locomotion. We do not place conscious effort into thinking about the sequence of muscles required to contract in order to move us towards the kitchen. It is likely that our conscious mind continues to remain focused on the intended goal, the food that initiated the movement. Whilst this is a simple example, this same process occurs on a bigger scale that creates our daily habits, beliefs and actions.

Our dominant thoughts about food lead to dominant feelings and emotions connected with food which impact upon our

Nutrition's Playground

actions and determine our results. This is the process that food manufacturers pay marketing experts to create for their product advertising. The more that they can create certain thoughts and stir up particular emotions as a result of advertising their food products the more they will increase sales because more people will act upon the thoughts and emotions they had. Food advertising often drives this process for both short and long term gain. They try to appeal to factors that will influence the impulse buy as well as creating long term beliefs and opinions about their company and foods that will influence buying decisions for a lifetime. Just like we have particular brands of clothing, electrical equipment or cars that we prefer or trust, many people build up a trust or preference for particular brands of food and will choose that brand over any other similar food product. The question has to be asked in generating food brand preferences: are we acting purely of our own accord or are we reacting to the marketing influences of a company that has consistently been presented to us over a period of time?

Marketing influences for each food product can come to us in many different ways. The larger companies may invest much in television or radio advertising, magazine and newspapers, public billboards, internet advertising banners, viral marketing, sponsorship of sport or television programmes, charity involvement to improve public relations, in-store placards, paid-for positioning on the supermarket shelves, two-for-one deals and even the food packing itself are all ways in which marketing can begin to influence our buying decisions. In this environment of constant bombardment of information and advertising we are constantly reacting by thought and often even emotionally to the way in which food brands and products are presented to us. The marketing that resonates with us will likely have a greater influence on us and affect our buying decisions. Hence the question of whether our food choices are a result of acting independently

Nutrition's Playground

or a reaction to things around us is an important one to answer. If many of our food choices are the result of subconscious reaction, it may be time to make a radical change and start to consciously make independent food choices that will benefit the rest of our lives. The famous self help author, Jack Canfield said:

'If you don't get the outcomes you want it's because you have not responded correctly to the events that have occurred up until that time.'

If Canfield's principle is applied to body weight, energy levels, or overall health and each of these are poor and not where we would want them to be then it is directly indicating that we have not responded correctly to events and choices that have occurred previously. We have to accept that if we are overweight it is a result of past choices that have been made that have influenced us physically and now affect us in the present.

Past, present and future

The human being is unique because of our conscious mind and our ability to respond to memory and to project our thoughts towards planning for the future. As a result of this ability we can be greatly influenced by past choices and occurrences and by what we hope to achieve in the future. Memories of choices and experiences from the past regarding food can have a powerful influence on our choices today whether positive or negative. The physical health and shape of our body today is a testament to the choices we made in the past regarding food and exercise. However, poor past choices and our resultant physical condition at this time do not need to continue affecting our decisions in the next few minutes, hours, days, weeks, months or years. Just because you grew up and your family made their gravy for a Sunday roast with gravy granules does not mean that you must continue reacting to their preference throughout your life. Just because your mother preferred a particular brand of chocolate as comfort food when she was feeling down does not mean that you must rely on this same method of dealing with your emotions when they are low. Past food choices do not need to dictate future food choices. The additional challenge is that over time choosing particular foods or brands causes you to become accustomed to specific food products. These habitually eaten foods provide a specific experience that may bring about physical or emotional responses that induce pleasure or comfort. Therefore it is clear that family traditions, learned habits, beliefs about food and the physical or emotional response we have to food can also greatly influence our buying decisions. Once again we may be making our food choices predominantly in reaction to the world around us even if we are being influenced by experiences of the past.

When past experiences generate vivid memories it is surprising the strength of the emotional response we can feel in the present. Cast your mind back to a particularly poignant memory in your life, a real high or low, something that stands out compared to your normal day to day living. Once you have decided on the memory try to bring to mind the circumstances of the situation, the day, the location, who was present, the environment, temperature, the mood and feeling at the time. Really try to replay the experience in your mind's eye. Seriously - stop reading, close your eyes and devote just one minute to recalling this experience.

Thank you for doing this small task. Now, I do not know what your memories conjured up for you, but consider the feeling you are experiencing right now or as your relived that memory. In almost every case a vivid memory will stir up the same emotions that you experienced when you passed through the actual situation. These emotions may have filled you with love, sadness, anger, fear or depression. Regardless of what emotion you experienced when you feel that emotion again it can be a powerful driving force of either positive or negative action, or indeed, even a lack of action and procrastination. The point is that thoughts lead us to emotions which in turn motivate our actions. We are so much more likely to act upon something when there is an emotional connection or driving force behind it. This is why many people think occasionally about changing their dietary habits and often do nothing about it. The emotions that are driving their eating habits are connected to the foods they have been habitually eating for years, not the foods they may need to change to.

Fear and love

Perhaps the two most powerful motivating forces are fear and love. Usually when motivated by fear we are trying to move away from something we do not want and when motivated by love we are moving towards something that we do want. When someone has been told by their doctor they need to change their eating habits because of the threat of illness, the primary motivation is fear because they want to move away from the risk of illness or disease. When someone gets real pleasure and satisfaction from enjoying a beach holiday with the important people in their life they will likely be motivated by love to make changes, eat well, lose weight and move towards looking and feeling great to enhance that experience. However, both these situations can be reversed and motivated by the opposite driving force. A sick person may longingly seek the feeling of being healthy and vibrant and, as such, is motivated by the love of good health, whilst the holiday goer may be motivated by the fear of looking bad in a bikini or swim shorts in front of other people. Remember, fear drives us away while love draws us toward. What do your eating habits say about you? Are you eating out of fear and moving away from something or out of love and towards something? Love is the more profound and influential motivating force out of the two, yet the most common motivating force is usually fear as people try to avoid gaining weight or getting sick! It is important, then, as part of dietary change to shift the motivating force from the negative to the positive.

In order to have positive motivating forces behind dietary change, the first step is to generate positive thoughts that will lead to positive feelings and positive beliefs. So what positive things about eating well can serve as the underlying thoughts? Here are a few examples to get things started.

Eating good food will lead to better energy levels consistently throughout each day

Eating good food will balance our moods and emotions more positively

Eating good food will provide mental clarity and the ability to focus when needed

Eating good food will improve muscle tone and function

Eating good food will normalise our body weight to a comfortable, healthy and easy to maintain level

Eating good food will improve signs, symptoms and feelings of health and wellbeing

Nutrition's Playground

Eating good food will improve sleep quality and lead to a refreshed and replenished body upon waking
Eating good food will improve the look and feel of skin, hair and nails

Eating good food will improve digestion and the health of the bowels

Eating good food will balance hormonal controls

Eating good food will improve our ability to cope with daily stressors

Eating good food will provide us with the nutrients our body needs for optimal function

Eating good food will balance our blood pH which leads to better cellular function and reactions

Eating good food will improve and balance our metabolism

Eating good food will, over time, lead to improved fertility, easier birth and healthier babies

Eating good food will lead to better dental health and fewer cavities

Eating good food will improve immunity and resistance to disease

Eating good food will improve the environment we live in

Eating good food will lead to sustainable farming and food practises

Nutrition's Playground

There are so many positive and motivating reasons to change our eating habits and move towards a more sustaining, healthy way of life. Perhaps some of the reasons listed above resonated with you as something you would like to benefit from and experience. Perhaps there are other reasons you can think of that are a higher priority for you to eat better and change your dietary habits. The key is that these reasons need to be motivated by love, a desire to move towards something and so should be thought about in a positive manner.

Sometimes we have been plagued by some health challenge for so long that it has exhausted our ability to be positive about it and we are only motivated by the desire to get rid of it, a fear of it continuing to negatively affect our life. For example, you are fed up with sleeping poorly, you are fed up with the constant lack of energy and you are fed up with the weight you are carrying on your belly or thighs. These negatives can become a heavy burden to carry when they are constantly viewed as a problem that needs to be removed, a health challenge that needs to be moved away from. Remember negative thoughts lead to negative feelings and emotions and as a result will lead either to inaction or unsustainable, desperate attempts to resolve the problem. These desperate attempts take a lot of energy and effort and usually have a short lived, minimal level of success. This can leave the individual drained and in need of comfort and recovery. Usually a place of comfort and rest involves a return to old, familiar dietary habits.

What do you really want?

It can be difficult to always know exactly what you really want. Over the years when I asked a client what they wanted with regards to their health and fitness, I have often found they proceed tell me all the things they didn't like and identified their goals through a series of negatives such as 'I don't like my wobbly arms' or 'I don't like getting out of breath easily' or 'I hate feeling so tired all the time'. We very quickly sense when things are not right and not in harmony with good health. However each of these negatives can be turned around into something positive such as 'I would like toned, firm arms' or 'I want to have stronger and better functioning lungs' or 'I want to feel more energetic and vibrant.'

Writing a list of things that you don't want can serve as a springboard for identifying what it is you actually want with regards to your health and diet. This may be a useful activity to engage in. Try writing a list of things that you dislike in your life that you want to change. The purpose here is not to wallow in self pity or to put you in a depressed mood, but to use your sharp sense of being out of alignment to help identify what it is that you really want. The vital and inspiring part of this activity, once the list is completed, is to take the time and turn the list of negatives into a list of positives. Once you have a list of positive items that you want in your life take the time to prioritise them starting at number one and so forth. Prioritising your list of wants will help to identify which of your goals will be the most important, the most rewarding, the most emotionally engaging and therefore likely to be the most motivating.

The concept of thoughts stirring our emotions which combine to bring about our actions should be well established now. There is one more aspect of this that must be understood because if it is overlooked it can undermine our chances of success. This process is often an unintentional 'get out clause' created by the mind because of limiting beliefs about our ability to succeed. The best way to understand it is by example. A very overweight person may identify as their highest priority that they want to be slim and attractive again, however almost in the same moment as setting this intention to move towards a positive objective their thoughts roll into the phrase 'but it is going to be really difficult.' There is a significant problem when a positive intention is followed by a 'but'. The 'but' phrase that follows in almost all cases negates the positive intention and shifts the focus and emotion away from the goal that mattered most. The 'but' phrase that follows provides a justification for future failure or low adherence to the actions necessary for success.

A 'but' phrase allows an individual to slip back into their old ways and actions that led them to being overweight in the first place. Then the individual will get more of what they intended, they will become more overweight rather than striving for the slim, attractive physique they set as their original intention. They have also protected themselves from the hurt and disappointment of failure by stating a belief about change that makes it easier to cope with. They decided right from the start that this change would be really difficult. When another failed attempt to lose weight becomes a part of their reality they are then able to soften the blow by saying to themselves, 'Well I knew it was going to be difficult, at least I tried.' When this situation is really analysed it becomes clear that the 'but' phrase that followed the clear intention to obtain a slim, attractive physique was the individual's beliefs about weight loss speaking out loud and clear. This individual had previously learned that losing weight is not an easy process, one that is very difficult to achieve for many people who are overweight, including themselves. Some find comfort in the fact that it is better to have tried and failed than to have never tried at all. Regardless of this, the harsh reality is they are still in the same place they were before they attempted to lose weight. Nothing has changed physically, because nothing changed from within.

Nutrition's Playground

A limiting belief may be created as a result of unsuccessful attempts to lose weight and so past experiences and the pain of disappointment has put in place a firm belief that weight loss is difficult and emotionally painful. Future thoughts, feelings and actions regarding weight loss are then constantly viewed through the filter of this belief rather than through the very reality that being slim and attractive is absolutely possible when the right actions are adhered to. The truth regarding past attempts to lose weight is that the methods or diets that were previously tried proved unsuccessful and weight loss was difficult. There is no reason whatsoever why the experiences of the past need to influence the current experience, especially if the system or actions being taken are different. If a new, fresh approach is being followed, then the individual has no past experience of this methodology and as such should not view future possibilities through the filter of past, unrelated actions.

Once again we see that a limiting belief is motivated by fear, the fear of experiencing feelings of pain and disappointment similar to previous unsuccessful attempts to reach a desired goal. So rather than being hurt, the mind puts in place some protective thoughts that shield the emotions against failure. However, the protective belief about change being difficult only serves to make this reality even stronger. Firm counterproductive beliefs reduce positive feelings and, as we have discussed, will decrease adherence to actions that will bring about change. The net result is the individual gets more of what they believed in. Weight loss will appear to be difficult just as they believe and they will continue to be overweight as a result.

Simply positive

So how do we set in place a positive intention without the 'get out clause' in our minds jumping in and negating our thoughts before we even get going? Firstly, we need to take our mind away from negative influences. So often the experiences of life drag us down to a level of complaining, gossip, tragedy and negativity. Think about the news, television programmes and the conversations with colleagues at work. Often these and other influences in life simmer on a negative level. Whilst it may seem unrelated to your beliefs regarding weight loss it is important to realise that negativity of any kind has a habit of breeding negativity in other areas of life. So it is vital to try and remove negativity from your life, even when others are just trying to be 'realistic'. What is realistic will depend on a person's life experiences. The individual who has become a multimillionaire has a very different, yet realistic view of life compared to the person who lives in abject poverty. The realistic view of those who have struggled to lose weight will be that weight loss is difficult and may not be possible. Whereas the opposite will be true for those who have successfully reduced their weight and managed to keep it off. It is also very common that we gravitate towards people who have similar views and experiences as we do and so we become supported in our lifestyle and beliefs by those who are on the same level.

It is very likely that there are those who currently influence you who will continue to support the views and beliefs you have whether they are positive or negative. It may not be possible to stop these people from influencing you as they could be long time friends or family members. They mean no harm and are probably completely oblivious to the fact that they may be reinforcing your 'realistic' view of life that restricts your possibilities of achievement. However, you are capable of redressing the balance for a time. You may be able to reduce the quantity of time you spend around those which limit your view of future possibility and spend more time around those who have either experienced success already or have a very positive attitude towards being successful.

Nutrition's Playground

Surrounding yourself with positive people will begin to permeate your being and have a positive influence upon you and will make a significant impact upon your daily thoughts and feelings. Consider those who meet together in weight loss groups around the country in a form of social support. Whilst they are gathered together in the common goal of trying to lose weight, there may have been those who have been overweight for years and are therefore holding onto stubborn, negative beliefs about weight loss. In many cases each individual will tend to relate and sympathise with the other members of the group and support each other in their belief that weight loss is difficult. Spending time with people who hold the same limiting beliefs will only serve to strengthen those limiting beliefs. In contrast, spending time with those who are a healthy weight, keep fit, eat well and are positive in their outlook of life will help to shift your thoughts and feelings away from the old, 'realistic', negative view towards a refreshing, more positive view of life and its possibilities.

Perhaps you feel that your current beliefs about life are well placed and very positive. A simple way to really review what your beliefs are deep down is to look at what you have brought into your life over the years, what is the residual effect of your long term beliefs? Are you happy? Are you in debt? Are you in a rewarding relationship? Are you overweight? Are you in good health? Do you enjoy food? Are you self confident? When we hold onto beliefs long enough they influence our thoughts and emotions and affect the choices and actions we take. Therefore, our beliefs very much bring into reality many of the things and circumstances we find ourselves in. If our current circumstances are unsatisfying or bring unhappiness to us, then we need to take a long hard look at our deep seated beliefs and how they are affecting our actions. If our circumstances are positive in some areas and negative in others then we may need to weed out the negative beliefs and shift them to fall in line with our other positive beliefs. What are your current beliefs, views and circumstances regarding food? How much time does food, shopping, cooking, preparation and eating take up in your day to day life? How much effort do you put into meal times? How much thought and consideration goes into purchasing food? How often do you eat fast food or convenience options? Do you ever consider the nutrient density or quality of the food you eat? Chances are your current actions and relationship with the food you eat says a lot about the beliefs you have about food. These beliefs can either be limiting or empowering.

Perhaps one of the most pervasive beliefs about food at present is that fat, especially saturated fat, is bad for our health and contributes to disease and obesity. This belief barely existed in society just 50 years ago, but today it seems to be touted universally from government publications to television cookery shows and everything in between. The strength of this belief has huge impact on the buying and food preparation choices that people make in an effort to keep healthy. This belief becomes so rooted in people that when scientific evidence is presented to the contrary to show that this theory has many flaws, as was discussed in an earlier chapter, it may have little effect on some, whilst others become very hostile towards the information as it shakes what was a very stable belief.

There are usually three ways in which people react to the opposing views that saturated fat is not bad for us, is unlikely to have any link with heart disease and should form part of our daily diet. A portion of people respond by completely discrediting the validity of the information, saying it is foolish or unreliable in order to justify to their own mind that their beliefs and actions regarding intake of saturated fat are valid and have so far been correct. Another group of people consciously understand the information and can see and accept that what they had understood in the past is much less stable than they previously thought and may even agree with the new concept that saturated fat is not that bad and should form part of our daily diet. However, this conscious understanding does not impact upon their subconscious mind and influence the decisions they make when purchasing or preparing food. Their actions continue as though nothing had been said or learned because their underlying beliefs have not been changed sufficiently to change their actions and long term habits. They may still harbour other beliefs that override the fact that saturated fat is an important component of the diet. For example they may enjoy the taste of the current foods they eat and believe that fattier foods will have unpalatable tastes and textures. They may believe that a change in their eating habits will not provide enjoyment and this is a powerful motivator in the selection of food we eat. An underlying belief about palatability sabotages the consciously accepted belief that saturated fat should be part of the diet.

The last group of people understand both consciously and subconsciously, right at the heart of their deep seated beliefs. This may initially cause a real shake in their beliefs about health and how to achieve it, but further research usually follows their initial shift and motivates a change in actions and choices' regarding their food. They benefit from the information they received because they were able to apply it to further study and thought until they began to feel emotive enough about it and act upon it.

Absolutely accountable

An absolutely essential part of making a positive change in our own lives is to accept that we are responsible or accountable for everything we currently have in life. Yes, I mean all the good things and all the not so good. This may be difficult to accept especially when it comes to our health and wellness. You may feel that by some unfortunate roll of a dice that life handed you a condition or disease that you did not deserve or you became overweight because your body stopped working right and your metabolism slowed down or your parents eating habits had become too ingrained by the time you began to realise that it wasn't that healthy. Whatever the reason you have learned to believe, the point is that you are looking elsewhere to attribute the cause, looking outside of yourself. It may feel easier to find an external cause or someone else to blame because it takes accountability away from us. However, by taking accountability away we also take away our power of choice and the ability to think, feel and act in a different direction. It is important to know and understand that we always have a choice and the ability to act in a particular way no matter the circumstances. By acting in a way that is of our own choosing we will create a reality that is determined by ourselves and not driven by outside influences. I am not saying that other people cannot impact upon our lives, but I am saying that we can always direct how those actions will affect us by accepting that we are accountable for ourselves 100% of the time. When we understand and accept that lesson we don't need to pass through the experiences that may make our lives difficult or upsetting to learn this vital principle.

'When you get the lessons, you don't need the experiences.'

Consider the following situation. A woman begins to put on excessive weight during her pregnancy and is consoled by two of her friends who try to be empathetic and relate as they experienced similar weight gain during their pregnancies. After the birth of the baby the new mother puts all her emotion and love into rearing the new baby and spends little time taking care of herself because this is what she believes

Nutrition's Playground

she must do as a parent. She continues to gain weight in the post natal period and feels she has lost her get up and go. It is even difficult to muster up any energy to continue caring for her baby in the way she has done so far. A doctor soon tells her that she has developed an underactive thyroid gland which has slowed her metabolism and she will need to take thyroxine to boost her failing organ. Initially she feels a real boost from the medication, but within a few months she finds her lethargy and general malaise begins to return much to her frustration.

In this story the woman continued to look outside of herself for answers to her problems. She believed her weight gain was caused by her pregnancy and this was backed up by her friends' experiences who confirmed that this was a normal part of pregnancy. The mother really disliked the way she looked, but accepted that something else was the cause and felt she had no time to focus on herself. She tried hard to fit into the idealistic motherly role and love the baby that had been the reason she had gained weight and damaged her self-image. But you can't blame the baby, so it is easier to just ignore the problem and focus on loving and rearing the new born. The diagnosis of under-active thyroid seems to have come out of nowhere and the woman does not have any reason why this should have happened and so accepts that life has dealt harshly with her.

The pregnancy, her friends, the doctor and even life itself appear to have brought all these circumstances about. These beliefs have brought the woman into a place of inaction. She feels she must simply accept what life has dealt her. Having accepted the current situation her negative thoughts, feelings of helplessness and lack of action will continue to strengthen the situation that she is currently in. The situation can only be changed with a change of belief. Whilst the woman believes she is powerless no amount of telling, educating or

Nutrition's Playground

motivating is going to change things in the long term. As soon as she is able to shift her thoughts and beliefs she can become accountable for her life and accept responsibility for each change and event along the way from pregnancy to weight gain to diagnosis. Then the power of choice and action can influence her reality and move her away from the life she hates and create something better.

Perhaps on the surface this example seems quite tough to accept. The story is not meant to imply that the woman purposefully brought upon herself all the circumstances that beset her, rather she allowed the circumstances to come upon her because of particular beliefs and lack of action. Nobody ever sets out to gain extra body fat or to bring poor health upon themselves, but the beliefs that fuel our choices and in turn our actions or lack of action can indeed bring these things into our reality. Some beliefs are created in reaction to the beliefs of other people or other circumstances. This is a vital question to ask. Are my current beliefs and habits about food and diet a reaction to outside influences or created and set from within? Accepting responsibility for our beliefs is the first step to accepting responsibility for the reality of our current circumstances no matter how good or bad they may be. Our current circumstances are the result of our past beliefs and actions after all. If you are unsure what your beliefs about food, nutrition and good health actually are then take a long, hard look at your current circumstances in life because they will only reflect what you really believe inside. If you don't like what you see then you do indeed have the power to change it. Your past beliefs do not need to determine your future situation. We often define who we are by what we have done or achieved in the past. This can be very beneficial if we have achieved great things and have had productive habits. However, if our life has not been as positive as we would like we may currently be looking back and devaluing our true worth and capabilities. If eating habits, health and

Nutrition's Playground

weight have been managed poorly then you have likely accepted that this is the way you eat and these are the foods you enjoy. Changing your dietary habits can only come about if you become fully accountable for how you eat, put aside any excuses and work at redefining the beliefs that you have built up in the past about how you eat.

When will now be the right time to change your dietary beliefs and habits? Have you been living and eating in reaction to the persistent influences around you? One of the greatest gifts we have is our freedom of choice. But with great gifts or blessings comes great responsibility. Many people believe their freedom of choice allows them to eat as they would like - any type of food at any time. However, with choices there always follow consequences and we cannot choose the consequences. Consequences can be good or bad. Although it is not always a guarantee, in most cases good choices bring good consequences and vice versa. Choosing unhealthy, processed and refined foods, regardless of your beliefs about how food will affect you, will still result in poor health over time in the majority of people. Choosing healthy, natural foods will usually result in good health whether or not an individual understands or believes this to be so.

Whether your beliefs and habits surrounding food and diet have been positive or negative the intention of this chapter is to bring to the forefront the need to consciously take control and act positively in your eating and food choices. Only you can do it. Only you can analyse your beliefs and change them. Only you can make the choices that will bring optimal health and weight. The power needed is within. Seek it out and nurture it. Shift your dominant thoughts, change your limiting beliefs, build up positive emotions and you are certain to succeed!

Step 10: Thoughtful Motivation for Change

We have already established the inseparable link between thoughts, emotions and beliefs and how the actions that follow are always a result of these three powerful driving forces. Perhaps one of the most significant reasons why we slip or fall in our efforts to change habits and lifestyle is because we are conditioned to place most of our effort on the physical performance of the actions necessary for change. This is a little like putting the cart before the horse. Actions are motivated most powerfully by our emotions which in turn resonate with our dominant thoughts and beliefs. If our thoughts, beliefs and emotions are not in alignment with our actions we have created a recipe for failure even if the actions being taken are positive. Incongruent thoughts and beliefs will slowly eat away at any efforts to change until the outward actions fall back in line and life returns back to the way it was before a change in behaviour was attempted. It is absolutely essential, therefore, that a change in behaviour needs to be coupled with a re-education of beliefs, a retraining of thought and a shift in our dominant emotions surrounding food and diet.

This chapter will provide a number of practical activities and processes that will provide indispensable help in the training of thoughts and moving towards a more consistent, positive emotional state with regards to changing food habits. These processes are not intended to be used haphazardly, but to be selected and used wisely in relation to your current or dominant thoughts and emotions.

Nutrition's Playground

Wouldn't it be nice?

This activity will be best applied when you are feeling discouraged, disappointed or frustrated in your efforts to change. When we are trying to achieve something new or different we often say to ourselves, 'I really want this thing to happen that hasn't happened.' This may be with regard to any number of health related intentions such as losing weight, increasing energy levels or recovery from an illness. This particular thought process activates mixed emotions because the thought has both a positive and negative side to it. The positive side is the desire to achieve this new objective, but any positive emotions that are generated are almost instantly neutralised by the recognition that you haven't yet achieved it. Rather than running thoughts through your mind about how much you want something that hasn't been achieved it is more conducive of positive emotions to take the pressure off and consider how nice it would be if you achieved something. Some examples of this way of thinking are:

Wouldn't it be nice if I was able to fit into that great new outfit I saw today?

Wouldn't it be nice if my stomach were more toned?

Wouldn't it be nice if I felt energetic all day long?

Wouldn't it be nice to feel emotionally balanced throughout my working day?

Wouldn't it be nice if I enjoyed meals that I cooked from scratch in my own kitchen?

Nutrition's Playground

These kinds of thoughts introduce a new perspective to the mind. Rather than highlighting the lack of achievement it leads to further thoughts about how and why it would be nice to achieve the said objective. By instigating a stream of positive thoughts it begins to shift us towards more upbeat emotions. Initially it may work more effectively to write these 'Wouldn't it be nice...' statements down on a piece of paper rather than to just run them through your mind. Writing things down requires more time and attention than simply flashing a thought across your mind. You will find you ponder over the thoughts more as you pen them on a page. A little practice with this activity will soon lead to the point where just stopping and taking a little time to run the process through your mind will be enough to improve your emotional state.

Better thoughts

This activity is best applied when you are feeling angry, discouraged, overwhelmed or you find yourself blaming others for current circumstances. The basis for this activity is in understanding that every objective really has two sides to it. The recognition that you desire something and the absence of the thing you desire. These different sides to each goal carry with them very different emotional frequencies. Pondering over something you desire can have very positives effects, but if your thoughts slip over to the other side and the current absence of the thing you desire this will shift your feelings to more negative ones. Often the things we want most become the things we talk about most often. Have you noticed that those who have poor health talk a lot about their illness and their efforts to get better? Those who want to lose weight constantly talk about their latest diet. Those suffering from lack of energy constantly identify how tired they feel and want to find more energy. Their desire to have this 'want'

Nutrition's Playground

is so high that it becomes a key topic of conversation in their lives, but they don't realise that every subject has two sides, what they want and the lack of it. Although much of their conversation is about what they want, if this objective is not being achieved it is because they are unintentionally focusing more on the lack of what they want. It may be hard to identify the difference because thoughts can flash across our minds so quickly. The way to know and learn the difference is to pay attention to how you feel in relation to the thoughts you are having. It is usually best to do this activity when something negative has happened that offers resistance to what it is that you want. Initially it would be best to write your thoughts down as it provides more time to ponder each thought and consider how it is making you feel.

The basic idea is to write down how you are currently thinking and feeling regarding a topic or situation that has recently happened. Next write another statement that expands or amplifies the first statement. Once you have written a few statements that clearly identify how you feel and describe your current emotional frequency try to reach for some thoughts that feel just a fraction better than where you are now regarding the same subject. After writing this new statement evaluate whether that thought feels better, worse or the same as the initial feelings described in your starting statements. Imagine that you have been trying to lose weight and you are on your way home after a particularly bad day at work and whilst stopping at the service station you pick up a bar of chocolate and bag of crisps and promptly eat them on the rest of the way home. This activity after such an event may run something like this.

I can't believe I just ate all that junk, I am such an idiot.

I have so little willpower

257

Nutrition's Playground

Why can't I just stick to this diet and lose this weight I hate so much?

Having written the initial statements it is now important to strive for better thoughts and evaluate each thought after writing it. It is important that each new thought is only a fraction better than the last in order to nudge yourself in the right direction. When you're feeling negative trying to make a huge jump to happy and rewarding thoughts will feel false and only highlight the large gap between how you are feeling now and where you want to be.

Well it had been a tough day today. I was tired and deserved a snack. (better)

But I didn't need to eat all that junk. I should have chosen something healthy. (worse)

I have blown the diet now I might as well kick back and have a pizza and ice cream. (worse)

It's not that bad really. Come on, pull yourself together. (better)

It was only a small treat. I can eat a healthy meal tonight. (same)

My partner loves the healthy chicken supreme I can cook from scratch. (better)

I will feel so much better once I have cooked and eaten this good meal. (better)

There are no right and wrong answers to this activity. Only you know how different thoughts make you feel. It also doesn't matter how long the activity takes to shift you into a positive mind set. Sometimes you will shift your vibration

Nutrition's Playground

quickly, in just a few statements, other times it may take a while. The key is paying attention to the direction you are moving whilst writing your thoughts down and seeking to move in a more positive direction just a little at a time.

The way you feel about something can have dramatic effects on the way you react. If you allow yourself to wallow in the negative feelings created by a situation, the actions that follow will most likely only serve to enhance those negative feelings. By learning to put aside guilt and blame and nudge yourself up the emotional spectrum to a better feeling, in just a short time you can be feeling more positive and are then more likely to take more positive action in relation to your circumstances. If you change the way you look at something the thing you look at changes. As you practise this activity you will find in time you become much more sensitive to the feelings and level of emotion you are experiencing and will be able to run this activity in your mind rather than writing it down.

Finding a feeling place

This activity is best carried out when feeling pessimistic, frustrated, overwhelmed or angry. It is often the case that when we recognise that something in our life is not the way we want it, even though we may be able to clearly see want we want, our current situation governs the way we feel and sets our emotional frequency. This is because as we consider both thoughts, the current situation and the situation we want, the feelings elicited by our current situation far outweigh any fleeting thoughts or feelings generated by occasional thoughts focused on the circumstances we actually want. Sometimes people use the term 'find your happy place'. This usually involves a little imagination to conjure up some setting or experience that is desirable and would be enjoyable for you. Often people imagine a location, a holiday experience, a happy memory or an experience with others. Finding a feeling place is all about using imagination in a more directed manner. The purpose is to sit peacefully for a few minutes and to see yourself in your mind's eye as having already achieved or reached the goal or objective that you desire as though it is your present reality. Whilst you visualise the goal as though it has already happened it will shift your thoughts and emotions to a more rewarding place and draw you away from the feelings of absence or lack that occur when we focus on what is yet to be.

It is important that when you seek a better feeling place in your mind's eye that it is not a brief thought. Linger for some time in your imagination and try to focus on the details and feelings that are present in this ideal situation. Let's say it's the beginning of a new day and as you climb out of bed you perform your weekly ritual of standing on the scales. This time they show an increase of 2 pounds. A result like that has the potential to ruin your whole day if you allow it to determine your point of emotional frequency. Instead of getting frustrated about putting weight on and experiencing negative emotions that are only going to serve to bring more weight gain into your life you can shift your emotions by finding a feeling place that is better than where you currently are. Close your eyes and visualise waking up in the morning feeling refreshed and vibrant and ready for the new day. As you walk into the bathroom you don't even give the scales a second thought because as you look at yourself in the mirror you see a healthy individual who is an ideal body weight, with a smile on their face. Your energy levels are high, your mind is clear, you feel confident about how you look and now look forward to facing the world each day slimmer, vibrant and healthy!

Nutrition's Playground

The difference in this situation is choosing whether to react to the circumstances that were presented before you or to choose a better way. By proactively choosing to stop and visualise a better feeling place you can set yourself up for a much more positive experience and will then be able to respond to your improved emotional frequency with more positive actions throughout the remainder of the day.

Sliding up the emotional scale

This final emotional activity is useful for when your emotions are somewhere between despair, fear, depression and anger. Sometimes when we are in a state of negative emotion it can be very difficult to state with any clarity what the emotion that we are experiencing is. We just know that it is not good and that we don't want to be feeling the way that we currently are right now. In order to move away from a negative emotional state we first need to identify where we currently are and then strive to move to a new place. If you are suffering from an illness and feeling helpless as a result you probably want nothing more than to be healthy again. However, you are not going to travel from a place of sickness to a place of health, but from a place of fear of what may happen to a place of confidence in your health. If you are heavily overweight the answer is not just to move from a place of being fat to a place of being slim, but more to do with moving from a position of self-loathing and insecurity to a position of contentment and happiness. When we recognise the emotional shift that is required alongside the physical changes that need to take place then we can have more control in bringing the physical change into reality. Rather than wait for the passage of time that will inevitably be required to bring about the physical reality we can work on shifting our emotions towards the positive and use higher emotions to lead our actions more quickly in the direction of

Nutrition's Playground

the physical reality. The following represents a guide to our emotions in order from the best feelings to the worst.

Joy/ empowerment/ love/ appreciation
Passion
Enthusiasm/ eagerness/ happiness
Positive expectation/ belief
Optimism/ Hopefulness
Contentment/ satisfaction
Boredom
Pessimism
Frustration/ impatience/ irritation
Overwhelmed/ Disappointment
Doubt/ worry
Blame/ Discouragement
Anger/Revenge
Hatred/ rage/ jealous
Insecurity/ guilt/ unworthiness
Fear/ grief/ depression/ despair

Experiencing negative emotions elicits feelings of resistance and restriction that usually inhibit our actions and prevent positive movement forwards. The purpose of this activity is to make verbal statements or to write statements down in order to find some relief from your current emotional resistance. It is important to try and form statements that you can relate to that are better than where you are currently at, but not too far up the scale that it creates an impossible divide that is too far to jump. It is not necessary to jump from a negative feeling to a positive one, but to gradually move up the scale. If your feeling is one of insecurity then anger is a step forward; if you are feeling discouragement then being overwhelmed is a shift in the right direction. By understanding the sliding scale of emotions it is possible to slowly guide yourself up the scale to a better feeling place. If your negative emotions have set in only recently then it will likely be an easier process to move forward. If the negative feelings have been with you for some time it may take more time to shift your emotional frequency forward, maybe only a single emotion up the scale as each new day begins.

For example, if you have determined clearly that your emotional state has been one of guilt for falling into the same state of ill health that beset your mother, then you already know that the aim is to shift up the scale to achieve a feeling of hate, rage or jealousy. On face value this sounds like an unusual shift, but it is moving you emotionally in the right direction. The following statements provide an example of how this activity might play out over a few days

I hate this illness, it stole my mother away from me and now it is trying to take me too. (Hatred)

I am so angry with myself for not learning from my mother's experience and trying harder to stay healthy. (Anger)

It is my doctor's fault. An early diagnosis could have made a huge difference in managing this illness. (Blame)

I honestly don't know if I can manage this illness and head back to good health. (Doubt)

This is too much for me to handle alone. I need someone else to help me out. (Overwhelmed)

I wish I would just get off my backside and do something about it. (Impatience)

It's just typical. This type of thing always happens to me. (Pessimism)

Nutrition's Playground

I really don't enjoy the day to day management of my diet and medication, it's so dull. (Boredom)

I guess I can accept my current situation and just get on with it. Many people are experiencing much worse. (Satisfaction)

You know if I just try my best I am sure I can make some difference to my health. (Optimism)

I know that I can be healthy again as I apply myself in positive steps and goal setting. (Belief)

It is clear from this example that through a series of directed thoughts or statements you can carefully shift your emotional frequency one step at a time in the right direction. When we are feeling negative it is sometimes difficult to know how to get out of the current feeling place. We usually just know that we want to feel good. By understanding the sliding scale of emotions we can in an organised and directed manner move our emotions gradually up the sliding scale to a place of positive emotional wellbeing where our further thoughts, feelings and actions are going to be constructive and beneficial.

Now that we have discussed a number of processes for shifting your dominant thoughts and feelings in a more positive direction, it is also important to have a few practical suggestions for helping you move forward in your food choices.

The best of the worst

Despite all our best efforts to be organised and plan ahead, there are times when you simply need to eat and, darn it, there just isn't a local, organic farm shop to hand to satisfy

Nutrition's Playground

your needs. A typical example of this is when you are travelling on a long journey and you need to stop and have a snack to maintain your blood sugar in order to be able to continue driving and keep focused while at the wheel of your car. In an ideal world you may have prepared some healthy snacks and brought them in advance on the journey for just such a reason. However, this is not always possible. Unfortunately the roadside services and rest stops only tend to provide a selection of foods of low quality and little nutritional value at heavily inflated prices. Often in these situations people just accept their apparent circumstances and put little effort into finding something of nutritional value. It is easy to justify that there is little choice but to eat the poor quality food on offer. This can cause three different things to happen. First, you change your emotional set point down the scale because you have had to go against your better judgement concerning food and give in to something of poor quality to eat. Second, you may find it frustrating to pay higher prices for poor quality food, which also shifts your emotional set point down the scale. Finally the food that is eaten has little positive effect on your energy and metabolism and so after a short lift it usually begins to have less than positive physical effects which may leave you feeling irritable, moody and tired. Not really an ideal state to continue a long journey. All in all it has not turned out to be a positive experience.

In this situation it is wise to apply the attitude of finding the best of the worst. Whilst the overall quality and nutrient density is less than ideal, you can salvage some benefit by keeping closer to your chosen path and using your power of discernment and choice to select the best foods that are available. It may take a little practise to learn which foods in these settings may provide some level of nutritional quality. By considering how each food is going to physically affect you and choosing those that will provide some sense of balance it is more likely you will feel more sustained later on in your journey. A simple yet effective consideration to remember is to eat some protein as part of the snack. This will help sustain a sense of satisfaction and will keep blood sugar elevated for much longer than a cheap, predominantly carbohydrate snack. It is also important to know you are using your power of choice rather than being forced upon by your circumstances to make a choice you do not want to make. By using good judgement and buying the best of the worst available you will leave in a better emotional place knowing that you still retained some control of your circumstances and came out on top. We are told that success breeds success. By choosing the best of what is available in more difficult circumstances it can help maintain a positive view of your food habits which will make it easier the next time a less than ideal food choice presents itself.

The next best thing

This activity is a great help during the transition towards a better quality, nutrient dense diet. There is nothing complex about carrying out this process as the name probably provides enough information by itself to teach the concept. The idea is that when you are doing the weekly shopping to set a target of how many foods you can change during the shop to buy the next best thing. It would probably be too time consuming and probably quite expensive to make the jump to the next best food item for everything in your shopping basket. I suggest that you start with a manageable goal of 5 items at a time. If you normally purchase the ground minced beef found in the frozen food section you may decide as part of your first shopping trip to shift up one quality point and buy the fresh value mince instead. It is important for this change to feel like it is part of the normal routine before you

Nutrition's Playground

shift again up the scale to buy better quality steak minced beef. This will later lead to free range steak mince and then to organic, free range steak mince. Making too many jumps up the scale before the change has become a habit can begin to offer a sense of resistance because it starts to feel foreign to previously established habits. Allowing yourself a period of time to gradually work each change into your normal routine will bring a sense of consistency and permanence. Striving for the next best thing across just 5 items at a time seems easier to manage and also provides some momentum to the direction you are headed as dietary change becomes an accepted part of your regular actions towards goal achievement.

These various activities are designed to assist you in developing your strength of motivation through shifting your emotional frequency and resultant actions in the right direction. This is an absolutely essential part of the success equation in the long term. Many have succeeded through pure will power and determination to change their health or weight for a period of time, but without shifting the underlying beliefs and emotions it becomes a challenge to sustain the change. When our thoughts and beliefs are in alignment with our current actions and both resonate together, then you are assured of your new path and the change will become a more permanent feature in your life. Guiding our thoughts and emotions towards a more positive state will make it possible to retain a higher level of determination and self accountability. There is something uniquely rewarding about developing our understanding, then applying this new found knowledge with determination and finally observing success as the outcome. The process of change does not need to be a challenge, but a rewarding journey of self discovery. In this particular case where the changes are dietary the rewards of improved health and vitality are more than worth every effort that is invested.

Nutrition's Playground

Conclusion

The hard work has come to an end. The ten steps of the slide in Nutrition's playground have been climbed with each chapter you have read. The journey has required a reasonable amount of effort and determination on your part and now, in position at the top of the slide you have a much improved perspective on the world of nutrition and diet. Some myths have been exposed and the real nature of food and optimal health has been laid out in front of you. You can see the slide clearly. You understand what is required in order to bring health, strength and vitality into your life. Now it is time to sit down, make the changes necessary and enjoy the ride. You may have already started to apply some principles whilst you were reading the book. Perhaps you decided to wait until you understood all the information and developed a complete action plan to ensure your initial actions were the right ones. Whichever course you have chosen it is time to boldly say, 'Stand up, be counted! Now is the time for action!'

Many of the larger playgrounds or water parks in the world have long and winding slides. These slides are built from many sections joined together. Sometimes the slides are straight and steep, other times they are winding and twisty. Both ultimately offer a ride that gets us to the bottom. The information in this book, if applied appropriately in a systematic manner, can provide you a straight ride to health and vitality which, after all, is the most direct route. However, life usually tends to throw a few curves and bends at us and so the ride may not be straight forward, but just like the slide

Nutrition's Playground

with bends and curves, we will still make it to the bottom if we trust in the direction it is taking us and stay on the slide. You will likely determine how straight or winding your slide is towards optimal health and weight by the decisions you make from this point onwards. As you now embark on a journey of change with regard to your food and eating patterns, perhaps we can discuss a few final tips that may make a difference in how you approach this time of progress.

Make a plan and write it down. This is probably one of the most important factors. Many people think they can simply mull over their ideas and that it is sufficient to know what they want to achieve in their head. We have, however, discussed the power of transferring your thoughts onto paper already. It takes longer to pen them onto paper which provides time to focus and ponder upon your thoughts and ideas. This will help to bring clarity and shift your emotions in line with your new positive thoughts.

Divide your ultimate goals into smaller, more manageable chunks. This is not only to simplify things a little, but to allow several stages of reflection between the start and final objective. By having checkpoints along the way it provides time to ensure you are still heading in the right direction, to regroup, to redirect your thoughts and align your emotions again for another push forward. Remember that change can create resistance and if we generate too much resistance because the changes are too extreme it may reduce our chances of success. Have you ever been on a slide and lost your momentum? It is not so much fun when you are going slow trying to push yourself forward. When embarking on a new path we often start with great waves of enthusiasm and plenty of motivation. We must use this early momentum to our advantage. Therefore, a solid foundation for action with

Nutrition's Playground

carefully planned review points can serve to maintain the pace whilst on your personal journey to health.

Focus on one dietary area at a time. If you feel that dairy is in most need of change then begin with this as a focus area. Whilst you may feel that you can do other small things at the same time, be sure to make your greatest efforts to shift from your current quality of dairy up the scale towards organic, grass fed, unprocessed dairy produce. After each shift in quality up the scale, change your focus to another area. Soon enough you will have shifted all areas of your diet from average quality to good quality. Then you can revisit the same dietary areas and shift the quality again from 'good' up to 'very good' and later on up to the best quality food you can find and afford.

Act upon ideas quickly. It is important to act upon thoughts and ideas whilst they invoke some emotional response in you. Usually when an idea first flashes upon our minds we think it over and this often leads to some enthusiasm. This is the time for action. I strongly suggest you do something that requires physical action and moves you in the direction of the new idea within 24 hours of receiving the inspired thought. Taking too much time to think it over, within just a few days, will cause a loss of initial impact and the emotion behind the idea starts to dim. Procrastination, as the word itself virtually implies, leads to *practically no action*. Early action, even just planning or investigating options, leads to more effective change and earlier goal achievement.

Last of all, enjoy the ride. It's a slide after all, it is meant to be fun! Discovering new food, learning to prepare it and most of all enjoying the experience of eating each meal should bring great fulfilment into your life. Knowing where your food has come from, knowing that it is nutrient dense and knowing it

Nutrition's Playground

will contribute to your health and strength only adds to the experience. There is so much to gain from a change in the right direction. The lessons have been learned, the tools have been provided, and now all that remains is for you to act. Follow your heart for the power is within.

'Take the first step in faith. You don't have to see the whole staircase. Just take the first step.'

Dr. Martin Luther King Jr.

Nutrition's Playground

Nutrition's Playground

Bibliography

Chapter 1:

Blythman, J., (2006). Bad Food Britain, Fourth Estate.

Blythman, J., (2004). Shopped, Harper Perennial.

Lawrence, F., (2004). Not on the Label, Penguin.

NHS Information Centre, (2010). Statistics on Obesity, Physical activity and diet: England, 2010, The Health and social care information centre.

Ogden, C. and Carroll, M., (2010). Prevalence of overweight, obesity and extreme obesity among adults: United States, trends 1976-1980 through 2007-2008, Centres for Disease Control and Prevention.

Chapter 2:

Price, W. A., (2004). Nutrition and Physical Degeneration, 6th Edition, Price-Pottenger Nutrition Foundation.

Chapter 3:

Albritton, J., (2003). Wheaty indiscretions: What happens to wheat from seed to storage, Wise Traditions in Food, Farming and the Healing Arts, spring edition.

Graudal et al, (1998). Effects of sodium restriction on blood pressure, rennin, aldosterone, catecholamines, cholesterols and triglyceride. The Journal of the American Medical Association, 279:17, 1383-1391.

How sugar is made, accessed from www.sucrose.com on 14th Jan 2008.

Nutrition's Playground

Lipski, E., (2004). Digestive Welness, 3rd Edition, McGraw-Hill.

Schmid, R., (2003). The Untold Story of Milk. New Trends Publishing.

Taubes, G., (2000). The (Political) Science of Salt, American Association for the Advancement of Science, accessed from www.junkscience.com on 29th Jan 2008.

The Salt Industry, accessed from www.saltinstitute.org on 29th Jan 2008.

Chapter 4:

Batmanghelidj, F., (2007). Water and Salt: your healers from within, 4th Edition. Tagman Press.

Beck, F. B. and Smedley D., (1997). Honey and your Health, Health Resources Press Inc.

Biser, S., (2005). The amazing health benefits of Celtic sea salt, accessed from www.naturalmatters.net on 8th Feb 2008.

Czapp K. and Ginzberg-Voskov G., (2003). Our Daily Bread. Wise traditions in Food, Farming and the Healing Arts.

De Langre, J., (1987). Sea salts Hidden Powers, Happiness Press.

Fallon, S., (2000). Fermented Honey. Wise traditions in Food, Farming and the Healing Arts.

Forristal, L. J., (2000). Maple Sugar – a gift from the Indians. Wise traditions in Food, Farming and the Healing Arts.

Nutrition's Playground

Gerez et al. (2006). Gluten breakdown by lactobacilli and pediococci strains isolated form sourdough. Letters in Applied Microbiology, 42:5, 459-464.

Graudal et al, (1998). Effects of sodium restriction on blood pressure, rennin, aldosterone, catecholamines, cholesterols and triglyceride. The Journal of the American Medical Association, 279:17, 1383-1391.

Mateljan, G., (2007). The World's Healthiest Foods, GMF publishing.

Rizzello et al. (2007). Highly efficient gluten degradation by lactobacilli and fungal proteases during food processing: new perspectives for Celiac disease. Applied and Environmental Microbiology, 73:14, 4499-4507.

Salts that heal and salts that kill, accessed from www.curezone.com on 29th Jan 2008.

Schmid, R., (2003). The Untold Story of Milk. New Trends Publishing.

Chapter 5:

Campbell-McBride, N., (2007). Put Your heart in Your Mouth. Medinform Publishing.

Dietary Goals for the United States, Select Committee on Nutrition and Human Needs, Press Conference Friday, January 14th 1977, accessed from www.anaturalway.com on 6th April 2009.

Enig. M. and Fallon, S., (2005). Eat Fat Lose Fat. Plume, Penguin Group.

Enig, M., (2008). Know Your Fats. Bethesda Press.

Nutrition's Playground

Enig, M. and Fallon, S., (2008). The Oiling of America. New Trends Publishing.

Groves, B., (2008). Trick and Treat. Hammersmith Press Limited.

Harvard School of Public Health, (2007). Low fat diet not a cure-all. Nutrition Source, accessed from www.hsph.harvard.edu on 5th Mar 2008.

Hicks, J. and Allen G., (1999). A Century of change: Trends in UK statistics since 1900. Social and General Statistics Section, House of Commons Library.

Kendricks, M., (2006). Statins and cancer. The International Network of Cholesterol Sceptics, accessed from www.thincs.org on 5th Mar 2008.

Kendricks, M., (2007). The Great Cholesterol Con. John Blake Publishing.

Luderin, (1999). History of Paul Dudley White. Journal of Interventional Cardiac Electrophysiology.

Nichols et al, (1976). Daily nutritional intake and serum lipid levels. The Tecumseh study. American Journal of Clinical Nutrition, 29, 1384-1392.

Ottoboni et al, (1992). The Food Guide Pyramid: Will the defects be corrected? Journal of American Physicians and Surgeons, 9, 109-113.

Ravnskov, U., (2000). The Cholesterol Myths. New Trends Publishing.

Nutrition's Playground

Sware, S., (2007). The big one – results of the biggest clinical trial of healthy eating ever. Junk food Science, accessed from www.junkfoodscience.blogspot.com on 5th March 2008.

Taubes, G., (2008). The Diet Delusion. Vermillion.

Chapter 6:

Argas et al. (1997). Low calorie diet. Journal of Consulting and Clinical Psychology, 64, 1-7.

Elliott et al. (2002). Fructose, weight gain, and the insulin resistance syndrome. The American Journal of Clinical Nutrition, 76: 5, 911-922.

Gaby, A., (2005). Adverse effects of dietary fructose. Alternative Medicine Review, 10:4, 294-306.

Kluger, (2007). The Science of Appetite, Time Magazine.

Taubes, G., (2008). The Diet Delusion. Vermillion.

Chapter 7:

Bjorntorp, P. (2001). International Textbook of Obesity, John Wiley & Sons, Heitmann, B L & Lissner L, Fat in the Diet and Obesity, pg. 137

Bjorntorp, P. (2001). International Textbook of Obesity, John Wiley & Sons, Pasquali R & Vicennati V, Obesity and Hormonal Abnormalities, pg. 225

Bjorntorp, P (1997). Hormonal control of regional fat distribution. Human Reproduction, 12 (1): 21-25.

Nutrition's Playground

Bray, G. A. and Popkin, B. M., (1998). Dietary fat intake does affect obesity. American Journal of Clinical Nutrition, 68, 1157-73.

Food Standards Agency (2006). FSA Nutrient and Food Based Guidelines for UK institutions. www.food.gov.uk accessed on 23rd Nov 2009.

Heini, A. F. and Weinsier, R. L., (1997). Divergent trends in obesity and fat intake patterns: the American paradox. American Journal of Medicine, 102:3, 259-64.
.
Hoare, J. (2004). The National Diet and Nutrition Survey: adults aged 19 to 64 years. A National Statistics Publication.

Howard et al. (2006). Low-fat dietary pattern and weight change over 7 years, The Women's Health Initiative Dietary Modification Trial. Journal of the American Medical Association, 295, 39-49.

Hulley et al. (1992). Health policy on blood cholesterol. Time to change directions. Circulation - Journal of the American Heart Association, 86, 1026-1029.

Hulley et al. (1994). Toward a more balanced cholesterol policy. Circulation - Journal of the American Heart Association, 90, 2570-2572.

Isganaitis, E. And Lustig, H. L., (2005). Fast food, central nervous system insulin resistance, and fast food. Arteriosclerosis, Thrombosis and Vascular Biology, 25, 2451-2462.

Lack, E. B., (2009). Fat metabolism and its relevance to liposuction. International Academy of Cosmetic Gynecology. Accessed on 9th Dec 2009 from www.iacosgyn.com

Nutrition's Playground

Pasquali et al. (2006). The Hypothalamic-Pituitary-Adrenal Axis Activity in Obesity and the Metabolic Syndrome. Annals of the New York Academy of Sciences, 1083.

Peeke et al. (1995). Hypercortisolism and Obesity. Annals of the New York Academy of Sciences, 771, 665-667.

Rissanen et al. (2000). A descriptive study of weight loss maintenance: 6 and 15 year follow-up of initially overweight adults. International Journal of Obesity, 24, 116-125.

Seaton et al. (1986). Thermic effect of medium –chain and long-chain triglycerides in man. The American Journal of Clinical Nutrition, 44, 630-634.

St-Onge et al. (2003). Greater rise in fat oxidation with medium-chain triglyceride consumption relative to long-chain triglyceride is associated with lower initial body weight and greater loss of subcutaneous adipose tissue. International Journal of Obesity Related Metabolic Disorders, 27, 1565-1571.

St-Onge et al. (2003). Medium-chain triglycerides increase energy expenditure and decrease adiposity in overweight men. Obesity Research, 11, 395-402.

Tunstall-Pedoe, H., (2003). MONICA: monograph and multimedia resource book, World Health Organisation.

Willett, W. C., (2002). Dietary fat is not a major determinant of body fat. American Journal of Medicine, 113 Supplement 9B: 47-59.

Williamson et al. (1999). Prevalence of attempting weight loss and strategies for controlling weight. The Journal of the American Medical Association, 282, 1353-1358.

Wilson, J. L., (2007). Adrenal Fatigue. Smart Publications.

Chapter 9:

Fortune 500, (2010). Annual ranking of America's Largest Corporations, accessed at www.money.cnn.com/magazines/fortune/fortune500 on 4th May 2010.

Hicks, E. and Hicks, J., (2006). Ask and it is Given. Hay house Inc.

Ray, J. A., (2003). The Science of Success. Sun Ark Press.

Vitale, J., (2005). The Attractor Factor. John Wiley and Sons Inc.

Vitale, J., (2006). Life's Missing Instruction Manual. John Wiley and Sons Inc.

Chapter 10:

Hicks, E. and Hicks, J., (2006). Ask and it is Given. Hay house Inc.

Ray, J. A., (2003). The Science of Success. Sun Ark Press.

Vitale, J., (2005). The Attractor Factor. John Wiley and Sons Inc.

Vitale, J., (2006). Life's Missing Instruction Manual. John Wiley and Sons Inc.

Nutrition's Playground

About the author

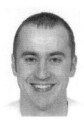 From his earliest memories Ben has been involved in food and nutrition. He always helped out in the kitchen as a young boy because he quickly realised that to enjoy food meant you needed to be able to prepare good food. This interest carried on throughout school and university and then served well as a support to a career in health, fitness and personal training. After many years assisting others to meet their fitness objectives, Ben moved into the field of education, working for one of the UK's leading health and fitness training providers. This served as a springboard for study and research, especially in the fascinating world of food and nutrition. The diversity of opinions within nutritional science spurred him into research, investigation and application with his family, friends and even the students he taught.

Ben is a qualified sports scientist, personal trainer, and metabolic typing advisor and is nearing completion of his masters degree in holistic nutrition. Ben has presented both nationally and internationally on a wide variety of subjects across both fitness and nutrition.

Ben is married and is the proud father of 4 beautiful and healthy children who have greatly benefitted from the traditional wisdom and health promoting capacity of nutrient dense foods.

Ben has also created a unique online resource for seeking out suppliers of nutrient dense, high quality food products within the United Kingdom. This can be found at

www.naturalfoodfinder.co.uk